Forties ON FIRE

HONOR YOUR MOODS
REDISCOVER YOUR SEXUALITY
THRIVE THROUGHOUT YOUR 40S

KATHRYN KOS

Forties on Fire: Honor Your Moods, Rediscover Your Sexuality, and Thrive Throughout Your 40s

Disclaimer: This book is not intended as a substitute for medical advice. Please consult your physician in matters relating to your health, particularly with respect to any symptoms that may require diagnosis or medical attention.

Publishing services provided by 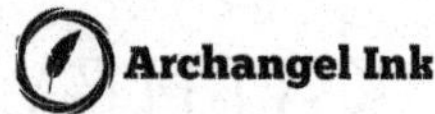

ISBN: 978-1-7307-0915-9

YOUR FREE RESOURCE

Before you begin reading this book, I have a free bonus to offer you!

In addition to the information already provided in this book, I have created a guide for playing! As adults, we still need to let loose, have fun and play, and in this guide, I'll teach you why.

To receive your free bonus content, sign up for my mailing list by visiting:

http://primalmusings.com/timeforplay

By signing up you will also be notified of any pending book releases or updated content and be first in line for exclusive deals and future book giveaways.

Immediately after signing up you'll be sent an email with access to the bonus.

–Kathryn Kos

CONTENTS

INTRODUCTION

"I just feel fatigued and moody all the time, and I'm becoming angry and resentful toward the people I'm supposed to love."

A client once said these words to me, and I've never forgotten them. Unfortunately, my client isn't alone in her experience. All too often women going through perimenopause encounter it as a negative season in their lives.

What Is Perimenopause?

As women enter their forties, they are usually unaware that PMS can rear its ugly head stronger than ever. We hear all about hot flashes and night sweats that will eventually happen as estrogen leaves our body in our later years. However, we don't really hear much about *perimenopause*. Many of us are quite unaware that our mid-thirties and forties can be a rocky and transitional time as well. Estrogen is leaving the body, and this can lead to strong physical and emotional changes during those years. For some women it can even start in their thirties with changing cycles and moods.

How can we combat feeling these strong surges of emotion coupled with fatigue?

Perimenopause Can Feel Like a Second Puberty

Many of us begin to struggle with mood swings, decreased sex drive, weight gain, irritability, fatigue, sore breasts, and acne—especially around our cycle. It can get ugly if we don't have the tools to support ourselves through this time.

I believe hitting our mid-thirties to early forties can be similar to hitting puberty for a second time. I've had clients tell me they feel like an angry teenager again. One particular client stated she felt a great sense of disconnection from people in her life. These hormonal changes can impact all areas of life, including personal relationships and careers. We may begin to reassess our values and try to discover deeper life-meaning. All of this is happening for us, not to us; and we can discover deeper truths about ourselves during this time.

Many of us are *just* starting to have children in our forties, and we want to have energy and feel good so we can laugh and play and enjoy our time with them. We want to feel the same way we did in our younger years.

To make matters worse, women often feel alone as they go through perimenopause. It's not something we talk about it. When we begin feeling "turbulent," our emotions are held against us. In our culture, emotions are seen as a weakness. Women are taught to be emotional, but not *too* emotional.

Ladies, I have good news for you: our feelings are our greatest superpower!

And you don't have to suffer through this phase of your life. There are tools and practices that will not only ease your transition through this time but can give you renewed purpose and pleasure. That's what this book is all about.

We absolutely can survive and thrive through our forties, feeling *and l*ooking amazing. The key is nurturing our whole selves, rather than cherry-picking diet and exercise (often with poor approaches, insufficient nutrition, and over-training).

Yes, life does get more and more demanding as we age. However, we can still have loads of fun! We can still have laughter, play, and sexual pleasure. We can feel good as we age. This doesn't have to be a turbulent time for us.

Finding Pleasure during Perimenopause

Diet and exercise play a key role in feeling good, mentally and physically, during this phase of life. However, these aren't the only factors. There are so many *other components* we need to consider to truly feel physically, emotionally, and spiritually healthy as we age.

We need to take the time to nurture ourselves, finding a balance in our moods and hormones. We can take the time to embrace our sexuality, sleep, sunlight, and free play. We want to feel good so we can be better for everyone else in our lives. There **are actionable steps** we can take every day to balance our mood, turn back aging, sleep better at night, have *real* orgasms, and maintain lasting energy without afternoon crashes.

My Role in Supporting Women through Perimenopause

Through the course of my professional life, I've worked closely with women and perimenopause for many years. I'm a Nutritional Therapy Practitioner with an M.Ed. in Rehabilitation Counseling. My primary clients have been middle-aged females struggling with hormonal issues and autoimmunity.

I take a functional approach in working with clients, as I believe it's important that we dig deep and get to the root cause of what women are experiencing in regard to their health. There are many terms for practitioners who search for the *root cause* and work with you to heal through dietary *and* lifestyle changes: functional medicine doctors, nutritional therapists, and chiropractors who specialize in a nutritional approach, to name a few.

Throughout this book I recommend functional medicine, though I am not a functional medicine practitioner. However, I believe with firm conviction that this unconventional approach works; therefore, I'm a big advocate. For many patients, there can be out-of-pocket expenses associated with this approach due to insufficient insurance coverage (the cost varies between doctors). If this is the case for you, I recommend finding a doctor who is open to exploring dietary changes, supplements, and lifestyle changes *before* turning to pharmaceutical options. Arm yourself with as much information as possible and be an advocate for yourself. Keep in mind that although there is an upfront cost, the cost of healing and feeling good without the need for multiple medications is priceless!

Most of us can agree that the state of health care in the US is scary right now. It's not really health care or preventive medicine at this point; we are *managing* masses of sick people. People who are seeking health, longing to heal from their struggle with autoimmunity, diabetes, metabolic syndrome, fertility issues, low sex drive, depression, anxiety, thyroid issues, and hormone imbalances. They are being put on antidepressants and medications. Yes, there is a place for this type of care. But all too often, traditional Western medicine relies exclusively on a medicine-based approach.

This paradigm is slowly killing us. Infertility is higher than ever and rising at an alarming rate. Autoimmunity and digestive disorders are rearing their ugly head in full force. I'm not writing this to be alarmist or defeatist. I'm writing this because I have some simple solutions for you, and I want you to take control of your health and well-being, rather than relying on a failing system.

The premise of this book is to support your wellness and vitality through this transitional time. If we can get to the cause of our mood swings, chronic fatigue, and low sex drive, making positive changes to support our *wellness*, maybe we won't need to be on so many different medications. The functional approach to medicine and nutrition digs much deeper, seeking to understand what is happening in the body and where you can make changes to heal. Oftentimes, a functional approach identifies necessary changes in diet, stress-management, movement, sleep patterns, and sexuality—to name a few. Practitioners take the whole person into consideration instead of singling out individual body parts. You'll find this is the approach I take in this book too.

I am passionate about finding ways to nurture the whole self: body, mind, and soul. I highly recommend finding a functional medicine doctor, especially at this crucial time when your body is changing once again. Stop brushing your health under the rug.

Functional Approach: Rachael's Story

Rachael is a forty-year-old mother of three. After each of her pregnancies, Rachael experienced increasing autoimmune-related symptoms. It started with joint pain after her first pregnancy. Further testing revealed a positive ANA test for autoimmunity, Sjögren's syndrome.

After her second pregnancy, she experienced increasing hair loss and greater difficulty losing weight postpartum. Prior to conceiving her third child, she was told that her follicle stimulating hormone was showing that she was postmenopausal (at thirty-six years old) and her chances of conceiving were slim to none. She was also told her FSH was so high that she would not be accepted into a fertility clinic. With the news of her infertility, Rachael and her husband began enjoying unprotected sex. Two months later she became pregnant. This made her realize that there is still much to be understood regarding perimenopause. Rachael obviously was not post-menopausal but, rather, was struggling with a hormone imbalance.

After her son was born, Rachael's autoimmune symptoms continued to worsen. She experienced increased hair loss, significant difficulty losing weight, dizzy spells, irritable bowel syndrome, joint pain, extreme exhaustion (she would "hit a wall" at noon each day), and difficulty with sleep. Even though she was attending CrossFit classes four times a week, she saw no improvement with her metabolic conditioning, strength, and energy. "I was out of breath and dizzy during workouts." She also experienced moodiness and irritability as well as irregular menstrual cycles.

About a year after her third pregnancy, Rachael went to her OBGYN for an annual exam. Her OBGYN told her, "You should probably start walking a couple times a week." Knowing this wasn't the answer, but feeling too upset to continue the conversation, she simply agreed with this doctor and left. It was at this point that Rachael sought out a functional medicine practitioner. As I mentioned earlier, functional medicine is an approach to that looks at the root cause of what's going on in the body, and rather than isolating body systems and treating each independently (typically with medications), the whole person is taken into account, analyzing factors like diet, lifestyle, movement, and sleep.

Rachael's doctor diagnosed her with extreme anemia, Hashimoto's (an autoimmune thyroid condition that affects millions of women yet often goes undiagnosed), low Vitamin A, low Vitamin D, iron deficiency, adrenal fatigue, and low magnesium. Her iron was so low that the doctor didn't know how she was even getting out of bed each morning. He worked with her to determine food sensitivities and helped her to make dietary changes.

Rachael's doctor recommended removing irritating foods from her diet and provided her with appropriate supplements to help with inflammation and increase her iron. Rachael took time each day to be outside barefoot and to play unstructured with her children. She also prioritized her sleep, making sure to go to bed early. Within a month, Rachael was seeing improvements with her energy level and joint pain. She was able to complete a workout without feeling dizzy. She is now two years into maintaining her protocol and continues to see improvements in her health.

According to her most recent blood work, Rachael's thyroid condition is fully reversed, her adrenals are functioning normally, and her iron levels are normal. She lost all of her pre-pregnancy weight and has ample energy at CrossFit, even competing in two weight lifting competitions. She now has energy to play with her children and spend time with her friends. She is no longer hitting a wall each afternoon, and her inflammation has improved drastically through removing certain foods she learned she was reacting to.

There are simple things we can be doing *every day*, no matter what our deeper health issues may be, that can have a HUGE impact on our physical, mental, and spiritual health—such as addressing our moods and mental health, moving our bodies, embracing our sexuality, getting outside and connecting with the earth, and cultivating the lost art of playing. We tend to focus our energies on dieting and taking supplements, which is a good positive step in the right direction. However, there are many more facets to health; plus, nutrition and supplement needs are very individual.

Although I will recommend some nutritional changes and supplements in this book, it's just one leg of the stool, and one that is unique to every woman. The other steps explored in this book allow you to take action *right now* to help you find balance and thrive through your forties. These simple actions can and will change your life for the better.

It's Time to Prioritize Your Self-Care

I'm sure you have heard this, but it's always worth repeating. When you're on an airplane and the oxygen mask falls, the stewardess warns you to put your mask on first *then* your child's mask. Why? Because you cannot help others if you are helpless. Oftentimes we feel guilty when we take care of ourselves or put ourselves on the front burner. However, if you are healthy, vibrant, and happy, you will be a happier parent, a more invested partner, and a better friend to those around you.

Think about it for a minute. If you're feeling miserable, how will that spill over onto those closest to you? How will this ripple out into the universe? By nurturing yourself, you are indirectly taking care of *everyone around you,* and even those who are not around you. We are all connected. Make sure you fill your own cup with all the self-care and nurturing you need so it can overflow and help fill the cups of those you love.

Stop waiting. Stop putting your health on the back burner so you can address everyone else's needs. The people in your life need you, but they need you to feel good and have energy first and foremost. Don't wait any longer to take control of your health. Being in our forties absolutely is a fabulous time! Start taking these easy steps right now, and you will be on your way to finding peace and balance in your life.

Chapter 1
UNDERSTANDING PERIMENOPAUSE AND THE HORMONE CONNECTION

Wait, What?

You may be saying: "Wait, what? I'm not in menopause yet!" or "I still want to have children! I still get my period regularly." And "I still struggle with PMS."

Perimenopause symptoms can actually start for some women in their mid-thirties, and the symptoms can be subtle to severe, depending on many factors. WebMD defines *perimenopause* as follows:

> *Perimenopause, or menopause transition, begins several years before menopause. It's the time when the ovaries gradually begin to make less estrogen. It usually starts in a woman's 40s but can start in her 30s or even earlier. Perimenopause lasts up until menopause, the point when the ovaries stop releasing eggs.* (WebMD, 2018)

Though this gives us a foundational definition for what perimenopause is, it doesn't give much insight into the experience of this season of life. The time of transition into menopause creates a marked change in the female body.

But does perimenopause have to be a *turbulent* transition?

A woman's forties can be an amazing time for her. It's a season of letting go of expectations and learning to respect her own needs. It's a time to experience massive emotional growth and learn to say no. It's in these years that a woman can really step into her sense of self, her desires, and her sexuality. We are, in a sense, *becoming*; we learn to own our true selves.

We *are* sexual beings, and that does not need to stop or go away as we age. Many women are choosing to start having babies in their forties and would like to do so without struggling. I love being in my forties! I feel a deeper understanding of my life, and I have a sense of purpose I wasn't able to find in my twenties or early thirties. We learn to respect our needs more, and we drop guilt and shame for not being perfect in all areas of our lives.

True, we begin to notice changes during this time, such as wiry chin hairs (ewww), acne, irregular monthly cycles, less energy, more fatigue. Many of us just can't party like we used to without a terrible aftermath. This certainly can be a time full of turbulence, waves, and strong emotions.

The Hormone Connection

Many of these changes have their roots in our hormones. There is typically a fall in progesterone during perimenopause, creating a dominance of estrogen that takes place around our early to mid-forties (Prior, 2005). Our menstrual cycles can begin to change as well. Our cycle can become longer or shorter. The phase prior to ovulation can shift, making our cycles less like clockwork. There are many claims that various supplements can balance hormones, and I will make some great supplement recommendations later in the book. However, don't forget that a holistic approach to hormonal health is the most well-rounded approach.

The first step is to know that what you are experiencing is the norm, though it may not be normal.

There are many factors that can contribute to an imbalance in our hormones. There are environmental estrogens (xenoestrogens) that can disrupt our hormones, creating a significant estrogen dominance effect (McLachlan, 2016). Typically before estrogen begins to drop, we experience estrogen dominance driven by a variety of factors. Our diet, stress (physical and emotional), environmental toxins, chemicals in personal care products, overtraining, repressing our sexual needs, lack of sleep, lack of play, and lack of sunshine—to name a few.

As a result, perimenopause can be a disruptive time for many women. To compound the matter, perimenopause is a subject rarely talked about. I believe perimenopause is not getting enough attention. When a woman gains greater awareness of this topic and discovers ways to support her experiences during this stage, the slow transition into menopause can become a much more peaceful and less turbulent time in her life.

What's so Bad about Estrogen?

Estrogen is a necessary hormone for many functions in the body, including glucose upregulation, immune health, and fertility, to name a few. However, what tends to happen is we have too much of a good thing. High levels of estrogen (estrogen dominance) during perimenopause contributes to many health struggles for women, including PCOS (polycystic ovarian syndrome), mood disorders, infertility, breast cancer, and other cancers. Estrogen dominance also plays a role in autoimmunity, which, for many women, tends to rear its ugly head after childbirth. We also have certain autoimmune related genes that may get switched on during a pregnancy.

Some of the symptoms of estrogen dominance include:

- Mood swings and irritability
- Breast tenderness
- Fibrocystic breast tissue
- Hair loss or thinning
- PMS
- Low libido
- Difficulty falling asleep and staying asleep
- Shorter periods or irregular menstrual cycles
- Fatigue
- Brain fog

Consider the following factors contributing to estrogen dominance:

- Consuming poor-quality food and processed food
- Using hair and skin products, cosmetics, cleaning products, and fertilizers containing estrogen-mimicking xenoestrogens (Watson, Hu, Paulucci-Holthauzen, 2014)
- Using prescription medications that affect the

endocrine system, contributing to estrogen dominance

- Experiencing falling levels of progesterone as we age, contributing to an estrogen-dominant state
- Paying inadequate attention to self-nurturing, sunlight, grounding, movement, play, sex, and nutrition

Working with Our Hormones, Not against Them

What are some ways we can work to balance our hormones naturally and, therefore, have smoother cycles? One often ignored action we can take is to respect our moods while supporting our hormones so we can have cycles that don't feel so much like a roller coaster. I believe it's important, first and foremost, to honor our emotions and not to write them off as "just PMS," or "just being too emotional."

You are not too emotional or too moody. The truth is, these wild feelings are there for a reason, and we need to acknowledge what comes up and make necessary changes in our lives, rather than sweeping our feelings under the rug. I believe this is the most important action we can take. Therefore, I will start by addressing moods.

You Are NOT too Much

You are a beautiful person who experiences different moods based upon your cycles, hormones, feelings, and stress level. Did you know that your moods are teaching you about yourself? How we feel does not define who we are. It's simply our innate self trying to tell us something that does not feel right. If you have not read the book *Moody Bitches* by Dr. Julie Holland, I highly recommend it! Holland shares some incredible insight on honoring our moods as we age, using antidepressants wisely, and navigating our changing hormones.

Holland states that we sweep a lot of "dust" under the rug, so to speak, throughout the first two phases of our cycle, the menstrual phase and follicular phase. During this time our hormones are more stable; therefore, we tend to let the little things roll off our back. When we stifle hurtful things and shove them out of the way, it just doesn't seem to affect us as much. This doesn't mean the feelings are not there—they just have not surfaced yet. This is because our hormones are more stable during these first phases of our cycle, supporting our neurotransmitters. The brain feels happier. It doesn't mean we aren't feeling anything. We just do a better job at pushing things away.

However, *after* ovulation, during the luteal phase of

our cycle, hormone levels drop, which also impacts serotonin (the feel good hormone) thus impacting our emotional health. We begin to feel more fatigued and moody, and we tend to have less energy during the second half of our cycle until menstruation.

Many women are treated with antidepressants (SSRIs) to help raise serotonin levels. While I think in some circumstances antidepressants may be warranted, I do think they are *extremely* over-prescribed, especially to women who are entering perimenopause and experiencing mood changes *due to hormonal shifts*. Going straight to medication without considering the wider roots of these symptoms does women a disservice. Rather than taking a medication as a *first* line, why not explore and address the root cause?

More times than not, doctors are prescribing antidepressants without truly understanding what is going on in the body to create these symptoms. Please hear me: **I am not against medication**. I understand that depression *must* be taken seriously, and in many cases antidepressants are warranted. What I am against is relying on quick fixes and BAND-AIDs in place of seeking a true understanding of the *root* cause of what may be happening within your body to create this imbalance.

The Luteal Phase: Work through Your S*&%

During the luteal phase, stronger waves of emotion come up. This is the time when the anthills become mountains. We may experience feelings of doom, darkness, despair, and sadness. You may be brought to tears over what seems like nothing to an outsider, but to you it feels like tragedy. We may get very irritable and testy with people. Before I make some recommendations for supporting yourself through this time and making it feel less rocky, the most important thing is to acknowledge the *messages coming from these intense feelings.*

These feelings are there for a reason, and we must experience them and feel what the underlying message is.

Our culture is one that chases happy and gets very uncomfortable with feeling any form of discomfort. We see sadness as a bad thing or as "wrong-feeling." However, "sad" is just as imperative an emotion to feel, even if it's unpleasant. Our hormones are sweet little messengers telling us big things, and we need to stop pushing away and resisting. Our solemnity, our cries, our intense emotions are needed in this world now more than ever.

In her recent TED talk, Susan David discusses the "positivity" movement, arguing that our obsession with positivity is a new form of moral correctness. We begin seeing people who are not happy as being wrong. Susan David suggests this is creating a "tyranny of positivity," and I couldn't agree more.

We have these emotional cycles for a reason, and these seemingly small things come up because there are things in our life we *need t*o address. As we age, those messages get louder. How many years have you been stifling hurt? What is the underlying message? Is there something that needs to be worked through? This is not a time to write off your mood as "just PMS." It's a time to sit quietly and feel what comes up so you can get to the bottom of it and begin to release the hurt.

Have that releasing cry. Have that important talk with your spouse or significant other. Talk with the people in your life about the things that are coming up and things that are upsetting you. Allow yourself to be vulnerable; nothing is off limits. Open and honest communication will help release any "stuck" areas in your life. Let those emotions roll as they need to roll, and try to let go of any shame you've attached to them.

This is a time to honor yourself. Honor your feelings. Respect your needs. Say no. Give yourself space. Give yourself permission to feel and express as loudly as you need to.

The luteal phase is the time for working through our shit! It's a time for going deep and learning about ourselves and our personal needs. It's necessary. Feel the feels. Work through the hard stuff. Don't write yourself off any longer. Stop stifling, hiding, and pushing away these important emotions. You are important; you are worthy of this.

On Shame

Women often believe that we are either too much or not enough. There is rarely an in between feeling of *good enough*. Since childhood, we have been socially conditioned to be "just so." If we express our emotions or needs we are labeled as "too intense" or "crazy," or "bitchy." If we withdraw then we are considered "unfeeling" and "stuck up." We have a hard time accepting the logic that we are always enough, just as we are. We need to hear this more often.

There is a lot of hidden shame that surrounds women and stunts our ability to be our fully expressive, unexposed selves. This shame stems from childhood and being taught that we need to turn ourselves down several notches to please those around us. To be ladylike. To be accepted. Often this shame surfaces at times when our emotions are running strong, and we have a hard time reigning ourselves in. This is reiterated when people look at you like you have three heads and do not quite understand why you are being so expressive.

Let it be okay when they don't understand. In allowing your truth to shine, you may lose people. Some people can't handle the true you. Those people are not *your* people, and that is okay.

Your people will see and accept you without judgment or expectations. They will stand firmly rooted with you throughout your wildest of emotions. If judgment or expectations are coming up, this is because something you are saying or doing mirrors an insecurity they hold in *their* life. It's always easier to blame than it is to look within yourself.

Embrace the glorious mess that you are!
—Elizabeth Gilbert

One important reminder (I have to tell myself all the time) is that how you are feeling does not define who you are as a person. **You are not your thoughts!** It's freeing to realize this. It's ultra important that we realize this. Those nasty little buggers that say terrible things to you all day long? That compare you to everyone else? That constantly scream at you that you are not enough and you need to do more and be more? Learn to recognize when you hear negativity in your thoughts. What kind of messages are you telling yourself throughout the day? Listen to yourself.

One technique you can try for combatting this negative self-talk is to journal through it. When something mean, hurtful, or negative comes up, write down the opposite of that. If you think *I should have done* ***that thing*** *better*, write down: "Wow, I took the time to do *that thing*. Good for me."

Repeat the opposite thought several times.
Remind yourself constantly that you are enough.
Hang those words on your refrigerator and mirror.

You are always enough.

This may take a lot of work after years of conditioning. But the more you practice, the more you can rewire your brain to switch from negative self-talk to positive self-love. And that will become a powerful transformative force in your life.

Shame from the past can rear its ugly head quite frequently. Shame can stem from childhood experiences, and it buries itself deep within your psyche. We tell ourselves the stories we have been led to believe when our young minds were being molded. However, we *can* learn to recognize these stories when they come up. Be an observer of these nasty little critters, but don't allow their false messages to take over. We essentially need to rewire our thoughts.

My therapist used an example of a car tire being stuck

in the mud and going back and forth in that groove, unable to get out. Once you are able to get that "push" out of that groove, it becomes smoother driving ahead. It's easy to continue sludging back and forth in the groove of shame over and over, letting it get deeper and deeper. It feels safe, and each time you roll it adds another layer of "stuck." It takes a great deal of work to push yourself out of the mud. However, once you do the work and get out of the rut, the road ahead is free and easy.

Each time you are true to yourself and your needs, you are giving that car a big push forward.

We have allowed ourselves to believe these terrible things for far too long. Consider another analogy: if you were to walk the same path every single day, it would become so familiar to you that you'd know every tree, every flower, and every bench. You could walk it blindfolded and still know where everything was. It's safe. This is what happens when we start believing stories we tell ourselves from a very young age. We blindly tell ourselves the same stories over and over, believing in these false truths about ourselves.

In seventh grade someone told me I had a big nose and that I walked funny. This led to beliefs and insecurities about myself that I carried into my adulthood. Maybe someone told you that you can't sing or you can't dance or you're bad at math. Our young impressionable minds take these false projections (fed from other people and based upon their own insecurities), and we run wild with them. We believe perceptions about ourselves that just *are not true*. These form our belief system about ourselves, and it's all a load of SH*T.

Find a new path to walk. Change the scenery along the way. Change the colors, flowers, and sky. Where you expect to see a muddy little puddle, instead place a pretty blue flower. You are a pretty flower just waiting to bloom. It's never too late to walk a new path.

Chapter 2

FINDING MOBILITY IN OUR MIND

Thriving in your forties, feeling good, and enjoying this season of life and beyond starts in the mind.

During a recent mobility (stretching) class at CrossFit, my instructor said something that really resonated with me, and I experienced one of those aha moments. We were rolling out our quadriceps on a foam roller, and she was talking about freedom in mobility and how it will affect our ability to perform better in all our movements. I thought about how having mobility in the mind would be freeing, not allowing ourselves to be tight and stuck in our perfectionist ways, but rather being more free and flexible.

How would we achieve this? As we rolled out our quadriceps and hit some painful 'hot spots' our coach reminded us to hold those hot spots for a few minutes and really feel the pain—then release it slowly. She went on to explain how in doing so we will develop greater hip flexibility and be able to perform better in all of our movements.

What if we allowed ourselves to feel and hold onto the pain that comes up in our minds for just a moment, and then *released it*? How would that free up our ability to handle all other areas of our life? Would we develop mobility of the mind? Would we perform better at life?

Absolutely. Yes!

Just as mobility in our joints helps us to become flexible, securing a stronger foundation for our body, so does mobility of our mind allow us to be more flexible in life.

Our external reality is deeply connected to our internal reality. Remember those lies we talked about in the last chapter? If you believe a lie about yourself, do you see it played out in your daily life? Imagine what will happen to your external reality once you begin to rewrite the story you tell yourself, once you replace those lies with the truth about yourself.

You become gentler with yourself, less rigid, less tight, more fluid, more open.

By not allowing ourselves to hold and release painful experiences, we tighten up and end up feeling stuck, following holding patterns, and being unable to move forward in our life. Remember the stuck-in-the-mud analogy?

It's important that we allow ourselves to feel everything we need to feel and equally important to allow ourselves to release it. In this way, we will possess the gift of *mind mobility,* and we will be able to free ourselves from those negative thought processes and patterns holding us back in life.

Thoughts Impact Health: Christina's Story

Christina is a forty-eight-year-old female. In her early forties, Christina was struggling with a Hashimoto's diagnosis and what appeared to be signs of perimenopause. Following a paleo diet template, she experienced some significant changes. She had fewer night sweats, regular and asymptomatic menstrual cycles, weight loss, and subsequent weight stabilization.

However, stress and her response to stress seemed to keep throwing her body off course. This became the most apparent during a time when she had to take on complex work responsibilities. She was telling herself that she was okay; however, she noticed changes in her skin, her cycles, her sleep, and her weight. The hot flashes returned. Christina cleared up her diet again, but it did not help as well as it had in her early forties.

Christina decided to add in daily meditation and made a conscious effort to let go of the noise she had created in her mind about who she was. She chipped away at the many layers of beliefs she'd formed through her lifelong relationships. As she dedicated her focus to untangling and rewiring her thoughts, she learned how powerfully they had been keeping her out of balance. Now at forty-eight and through this awareness process, she is noticing a physical improvement in her inflammation, cycle, stress, moods, perimenopausal symptoms, and weight.

The Mind-body Connection

Many people assume diseases run in their family and are therefore susceptible to whatever disease Mom or Uncle Joe had. Other people believe what we put on and in our body is the main culprit. Not many people are aware of or discuss the link between our *thoughts and disease processes.* Destructive, negative thought patterns can lead to disease processes in the body.

Gabor Maté discusses the stress and disease connection in his book When the Body Says No. According to Maté, "an intimate relationship exists between the brain and the immune system" (2011). Our response to stress contributes to disease processes in our body. He describes this connection in scientific terms as *psychoneuroimmunology*.

Our emotions throughout life interact profoundly with our nervous system, impacting our immune system, endocrine system, and hormones—at the cellular level. As I mentioned earlier, we like to separate our body systems and treat parts of ourselves individually. This is especially true in Western medicine. This may be a difficult concept to grasp, but all of the parts of us are actually one being. According to Maté,

> *Even to speak about links between mind and body is to imply that two discrete entities are somehow connected to each other. Yet in life, there is no such separation. There is no body that is not the mind, no mind that is not the body.* (2011)

Transforming Negative Thought Patterns

The following are some amazing techniques I recommend to help you change negative thought processes and catch that childhood shame when it tries to surface. Keep in mind, this is a transformative *process*, not an overnight fix. Neither is this a road to perfection. Let go of any expectations you hold toward yourself, and surrender to the process of unbecoming.

Journaling

Writing can be extremely therapeutic. It helps us to untangle the mess we feel when we are overwhelmed or unable to articulate our needs. Writing thoughts as they come in gives those thoughts a special place, a voice, a life, and an energy. It helps bring clarity. It can clear away the muck and replace it with answers. Writing is a great way to truly tune into yourself. It allows you to understand where you are placing your energy and identify what shifts need to occur. You can journal for as little as five minutes to start to see the benefits. Or, if you are anything like me, you might write for hours.

Listening to binaural beats with earbuds

What are binaural beats?

> *Binaural beats are auditory brain-stem responses which originate in the superior olivary nucleus of each brain hemisphere. They result from two different auditory impulses or sounds, heard from opposite ears. This binaural beat is consciously heard as the human hearing range is from 20-20,000.* (About Binaural Beats: What Are Binaural Beats Do They Work?, 2018)

Different beats stimulate different brainwaves. Beta brainwaves are the fastest, emitted when we are very alert and using a lot of mind power. Alpha brainwaves are slightly slower, occurring when you step out of a beta state to take a brief rest—to decompress and relax. Theta brainwaves are slower still and often occur when you are spacing out or daydreaming—think of that moment when you first wake in the morning yet are still in a half sleep. Finally, delta brainwaves are the slowest, emitted when you are in a deep sleep.

Listening to binaural beats has been shown to have a positive effect on creativity, attention, relaxation, decreased anxiety, and a happier mood! The best part is there are many different binaural beat meditations on YouTube, depending on the state you want to be in.[1]

Surrendering

Allow yourself to feel everything you need to feel: the good, the bad, the painful. We have become a culture very detached from our emotions. We are afraid to feel. We do what's easy and avoid the hard stuff at all costs. Stop stifling your emotions and sitting on them; instead, sit *with* them and befriend your emotions.

Do you find yourself reaching for things to numb your feelings? Things like alcohol, shopping, social media, or sex? Are you running away from your emotions? These distractions only stifle and build up tensions, creating more conflict in your life. Take time to feel what you need to feel. Those painful feelings are there to teach us so we can grow.

---

1 It's important to use earbuds when listening in order to get the full effect!

The pain is *temporary*. Once we feel it, we can release it and be okay. I recommend a very simple exercise:

1. Find a quiet place.
2. Put your hand on your heart.
3. Allow yourself to surrender your thoughts to do as they wish.
4. Then picture those thoughts blowing away.

Stepping away from Social Media

One of my favorite quotes comes from Theodore Roosevelt: "Comparison is the thief of joy." We like to make our lives look shiny and spectacular. We also love to compare ourselves to everyone else's picture-perfect lives.

Social media is notorious for contributing to this destructive habit. Social media is a façade.

We all have challenges we are working through. Every person has unfulfilled desires for more money, or a bigger house, or a more loving husband. It may look flashy and fun, but trust me when I say the people you idolize are struggling in one capacity or another—just like you. No one lives without struggle. We all struggle in different ways. We could all work on finding more peace and happiness in our lives.

Step away from social media periodically. Spend your free time with people you can converse with face to face. Practice being open and vulnerable with people you trust. This is an age-old, time-tested path to spiritual growth.

Chapter 3

EXCHANGING SHALLOW SPIRITUALITY FOR DEEPER CONNECTION

The Dark Side of Western Spirituality

The word *spirituality* is thrown around quite a bit now without a deep understanding of what it truly means to nurture our spirit. Regardless of what we believe about religion and spirituality, we are each on our own personal journey. Yet, we are all connected to each other. We often forget the *all connected* part, and spirituality becomes something glittery to show off and—once again—use for comparison with others.

Consider these phrases:

"Be positive."
"Vibrate high."
"Let go of what isn't serving you."
"Choose happy."

"Better things will come into your life."

These sayings are very trendy right now, especially among Millennials, and they typically accompany shiny smiley Instagram yoga handstand selfies. I think it's awesome if you can do a yoga handstand. In fact, it's a goal of mine! However, it's not a skill that makes a person more spiritual. This may be fun for the person posting online, but such showy displays that claim spiritual authority can make those of us who are still finding our way spiritually (most of us), feel like we've missed the boat.

I'm here to tell you that you haven't missed any boat.

Shallow social media–style spirituality is not serving human beings to truly grow together as spiritual people. What can we do about this?

Recognizing the Darkness

We must recognize that everyone is chasing after that elusive state we call "happiness," and it's all too easy to confuse spirituality with happiness. This is a phenomenon known as *spiritual bypassing.* Spiritual bypassing means denying any emotion that is deemed "not spiritual." We forget that *every* emotion that makes us human is important to feel and experience. Each one is part of our journey through the human life.

Yes, even the really difficult emotions guide us to where we need to be.

Spirituality is an outlet for us to find connection with others, an outlet that serves *all* of our feelings and emotions. It is a realm of peace and understanding and love. Every spiritual path explores this foundational dichotomy, whatever term you use for it: yin and yang, light and dark, beautiful and chaotic. Spirituality is a journey of discovering what resonates best in your world so you can better serve as part of a *community* and an integral part of the wider world—the bigger picture. In modern times, our conception of spirituality often ignores that community aspect. We tend to make spirituality about our ego. Community becomes a big missing component in our spiritual development.

The Western version of spirituality/personal development has a dark side. Avoidance of feeling anything other than "happy" leaves you feeling wrong, bad, or not enough. If you get angry, sad, insecure, or feel any other dark emotion that tries to surface, you've strayed from the path. This is simply not true, and it's a view that often leads to compromised health.

This can be one of the many reasons why women entering perimenopause do not talk openly about their moods and emotions. Instead, they are stifled or brushed away. We have been led to believe there is something inherently wrong with us if we are not happy all the time. We seek out medications, distractions, or anything to avoid feeling too deeply.

Do you find yourself judging people who get angry? Did you know that anger is a natural human emotion and a perfectly justifiable response to many situations? We think anger is bad or wrong, but it is a *completely normal* human emotion. Repressing your emotions so you can remain "spiritual" leads to inauthenticity, disordered thinking, and skewed self-perception. We begin lying to ourselves and those around us in order to be "spiritual enough."

Staying positive all the time requires you to bury things you will eventually have to deal with. You are here right now as a human. An imperfect human, not Buddha. Do I advocate sitting in misery? No. I advocate feeling the F*CK out of these negative emotions when they arise so you can truly learn from what is coming up. *Then* it's time to heal and let go.

In this way, feeling happy, "spiritual," and at peace with your surroundings doesn't become such a difficult task. And it's legit—not pretending to be happy even when you aren't and hoping your brain will somehow rewire. You can't feel and process the shitty things if you are putting your rose-colored glasses on 24/7. Life is not always rainbows and unicorns and sunshine, and that's what makes it so amazing.

Staying in the Light

As mature women, when we fail to feel "spiritual enough" we create just another reason to feel we don't measure up. I believe this chasing of happiness is creating a very sad, lonely culture. Happiness means finding joy in what we do have. Our real, in-person relationships. Even the yucky stuff. The hard stuff. The boring day-to-day monotonous stuff. And the things that just are not pretty, like our occasional adult temper tantrums. Out of my own personal life experiences, I've discovered that (as the saying goes) the grass is not always greener elsewhere.

You take the same shit with you wherever you go.

The secret that none of us know (because we are too busy chasing the elusive happiness) is that if we work on "feeling all of the feels" and learn to love the life we've created, it will open the door for so much more joy and greater life experiences. This is the answer. What isn't supposed to be in your life will fall away, and better things will come to be.

Paradoxically, it's embracing your darkness, your sadness, your negativity—taking the bad along with the good—that is the deep spiritual path.

Spirituality Is Not for Show

If you need to show the world how spiritual you are, you are probably still existing very much in the ego. Beauty doesn't equal spirituality, love, or happiness. We can find beauty in spirituality, but having a bikini yoga body, the ability to do a handstand, and beachy salty hair waves are not essential criteria for spirituality. The focus (especially on social media) has become centered around the ego, not around supporting spiritual community. The secret to happiness and longevity is community. We are social beings, not social *media* beings. Women, if you are not on Team Selfie, I promise you are still enough.

I want to talk specifically about the phrase "Let go of everything that doesn't serve you." This phrase comes in different varieties and gets thrown around quite a bit in spiritual communities. But the truth is: **Everything in life serves us.** The good, the bad, the terrible, the sad, the painful, the beautiful, the fun. It all serves us and helps us to grow spiritually.

Yes, sometimes we do need to let people and situations go. Sometimes we evolve and change, and we no longer resonate with the people around us, or we just find ourselves in completely different places. Sometimes we feel stagnant, realizing that something in our life needs to change. It is important to recognize this and allow ourselves to move and grow. Let go. Surrender.

However, other times we need to find the lessons in people and experiences, and work through these lessons together. If we let go of everything and everyone in life that feels difficult, or sad, constantly moving to the next thing and the next, we are back to chasing that elusive happiness again. We're little better than rats spinning in a wheel. When we go deeper and really look to gain understanding about the challenging people and situations in our lives, we can grow. That's where we find life's gems. It's about working through pain, and not always running away to what *may* be better. Chasing a high. Chasing what looks shinier.

Nothing stays shiny forever.

Women are now afflicted with trying to show the world how wonderful our life is. We're tempted to constantly seek external validation. The dopamine and oxytocin high we receive from social media validation can become an addiction. Especially when there are things in our lives that we just do not want to deal with. We are often left feeling dismal. We compare ourselves, feel inferior, and try to feel better by continuing the vicious cycle. We have become an instant gratification culture, and we need constant validation to feel good about ourselves and the world around us. We allow inspirational Instagram memes to guide our decisions rather than listening to our quiet voice within. This temporary high doesn't last, so we keep at it, perpetuating the destructive cycle. We have severe FOMO (fear of missing out), and have essentially become a bunch of neurotic happiness-chasers, running in a rat wheel.

We will not find God, love, higher vibration, or whatever we seek on our spiritual path if we do so in this manner. We'll find this deeper meaning through serving and loving each other, recognizing our differences, yet still coming together and accepting each other. We find our purpose, love, God, or whatever we resonate with through forming communities, inviting people into community, and serving others inside our communities.

How do we do this?

We open our hearts and minds to differences.

We cultivate the ability to see beauty in the small and simple things in life.

We practice more being, less doing.

We embrace stillness, letting go of our obsessive chasing.

Chapter 4
TOUCHING UPON NUTRITION

Having read that I am a nutritional therapist, you may be surprised that my main focus in this guide is not nutrition. Why not? The reason is twofold.

First, we are all different. We all have different biochemistry and dietary needs. There are so many trending diets out there, and it can be challenging to know what is best for *your* optimal functioning. It can be very daunting to find your way in a world where so many gurus claim their way of eating is the healthiest. Some of these diet paradigms are amazing and are truly helping people to heal. For example, I struggle with autoimmune conditions and have found that by following a paleo autoimmune protocol my health has improved dramatically.

When I was working with clients one on one, I admit I was dogmatic in my approach. I thought the paleo diet was the answer for *everyone*. In recent years, I've realized this is just not the case. I have since learned that different nutritional paradigms work for different people based on their bio-individual needs. It takes time to figure out what works best for you, but it *is* worth figuring out. With that said, my approach tends to be an ancestral health approach, with a focus on fresh whole foods, healthy fats, and sulfur-rich vegetables.

Making any positive change in diet, such as increasing real fresh whole foods and decreasing processed foods can create a great foundation for women entering perimenopause. Once again, I recommend finding a practitioner with a functional approach to help uncover the *root cause* of your health issues and find the best way of eating for *your* healing.

The second reason I am not focusing too much on nutrition in this particular book is that there are many other factors that strongly influence a woman's health. Many of these other factors are not talked about nearly enough yet are just as important (play, grounding, sex, sunlight, movement, and sleep, to name a few). As a result, it's these practices I want to emphasize in this book.

Balanced Nutrition

There are, however, several things we can do to find balance in nutrition so we can help make healthy hormones. Cutting out processed foods, sugar, and poor-quality fats, while nurturing our body with vitamin-rich healthy fats, quality meats (grass-fed/pasture-raised animal protein and wild-caught seafood), nuts and seeds, and dark sulfur-rich vegetables are changes that almost all women can benefit from.

Many of us are deficient of healthy fatty acids, and this contributes to a wide array of conditions. Women in our generation have become afraid of fat, due to the poor dietary recommendations of previous generations (based on flawed research). I can remember spraying a 'light' margarine spray on my corn on the cob, eating fat-free and low-fat everything. I can also remember that my depression and anxiety were at record highs during that time. I was essentially starving my cells of the nutrients they needed to work properly. Fat serves a great many functions in the body, and it's imperative for hormonal health and brain health.

Don't fear saturated fat. Eat fewer processed forms of carbohydrates. Eat *enough* carbohydrates to support glycogen for muscle recovery and sleep, especially if you are lifting heavy or working out intensely. My suggestion is to eat starchy veggies after workouts and in the evening. This is often called *carb backloading* and can keep you burning fat for energy yet give you adequate carbohydrates for recovery and sleep. Avoid soda, sugar, candy, and highly processed crackers, bread, pasta, cookies, and treats.

Most of us in the US are stuck as sugar burning metabolizers. We snack frequently throughout the day, thus keeping our bodies in a constant "fed" state. We tend to be on the infamous blood sugar rollercoaster, craving sugary foods and sweets throughout the day, often crashing in the afternoon with low energy and fatigue, relying on caffeine to get through the day. To stop the cycle, it's imperative that we decrease our intake of these unhealthy foods.

Rather than labeling and trying to follow a specific diet, you can start out by simply sticking with real whole foods, things that do not come in cans or boxes. And at all costs, avoid refined vegetable oils like canola oil, sunflower oil, and margarines. These highly processed oils drive up inflammation, the root cause of many modern diseases. If you decide you want to follow a specific approach (ketogenic, paleo, vegan, etc.) that feels right to you, do so under the guidance of a practitioner who can help you determine food sensitivities, genetics, autoimmunity, and gut issues.

Healthy fats help us to make healthy hormones. Fats

(the good kind, listed below) keep you stable and satiated throughout the day and are also great for brain health. It's finding the right kind of fat that matters. Some doctors *still* recommend canola oil for heart health, which is processed at extremely high temperatures and treated with chemicals (Egglezos, 2012). It's rancid and causes inflammation in the body. Avoid those highly processed liquid-at-room-temperature oils, and stick with:

- Coconut oil for cooking and baking
- Lard, bacon fat, tallow, shmaltz for cooking and baking
- Ghee for cooking and baking
- Olive oil, avocado oil, and macadamia nut oil for light sautéing or cold use
- Eat nuts and seeds soaked overnight and roasted low and slow

Digestion is EVERYTHING

We need to be able to digest and assimilate the foods we are eating. Unfortunately, the majority of us are not. Digesting food properly is how we get our nutrients. You may have heard the buzzword *leaky gut* going around in the natural health community. In a nutshell, having a leaky gut means the tight junctions in the small intestine (where we absorb nutrients) have pulled apart. This typically happens with larger particles of undigested or foreign proteins. Larger particles of undigested food and protein can pass through these junctions and enter the bloodstream. The body then sees these particles as foreign and mounts an attack. Leaky gut has been associated with immune-related disorders, skin conditions, and even brain conditions. Our brain is connected to the gut, and how we digest has a huge impact on our mental health.

What are some simple things you can do every day to support proper digestion?

- **Eat in a relaxed (parasympathetic) state or position.** We need to be calm in order to properly digest and assimilate our food. Make sure you are sitting down, not in a car and not during a meeting. Culturally we do not value our eating time. However, eating is a time to step back and away from being busy. Slow down and chew your food, savor it, and be thankful for the bounty in front of you. Stop rushing meals.
- **Chew your food thoroughly.** Digestive enzymes in our saliva help to break down some of the sugars in our food. However, when we wolf down our food and swallow large pieces, they become more difficult to break down during

digestion. This has a big impact on our digestive health.

- **Learn the truth about stomach acid and heartburn.** You are not making "too much stomach acid." Stomach acid is not the enemy. Do yourself a favor if you struggle with heartburn. Read the book The 30 Day Heartburn Solution by my friend Craig Fear. He teaches the truth about heartburn: you probably are not making enough stomach acid, and the foods you are eating are not digesting properly.
- **Work with a practitioner to identify foods you may be sensitive to, and follow an elimination protocol.**

We consume massive amounts of highly processed grains in our culture, and we trust and believe in government dietary recommendations. Grains contain anti-nutrients that can make them difficult to digest, preventing you from absorbing nutrients. Where has this gotten us other than on multiple medications? I do believe *some* people can handle small amounts of properly prepared (soaked and sprouted) ancient grains. Through soaking and sprouting, the food becomes easier to digest. Therefore, we are able to get the nutrients from the food without impacting our gut health. The problem is that people are not willing to take these preparatory steps, and we make grains a *huge* part of our diet. We do not take the time to properly prepare our food because we do not get instant gratification from it. We are busy and rushed.

My recommendation? If you feel you cannot fully remove processed grains from your diet, decrease the amount of grains you are consuming and stick with traditionally prepared ancient grains and legumes. This involves fermenting, soaking, and sprouting so your body can more easily digest and assimilate the nutrients. Gluten-free grains are easier to digest. I do not believe that going gluten-free is a fad. I've seen cutting out gluten help a great many people to feel better. However, if you can't part with gluten, I recommend eating fermented bread, such as sourdough, in small amounts. Why small amounts? Large amounts of processed carbohydrates raise our insulin and glucose, keep us as sugar burners, and affect our hormones, mood, weight, and health. Once again, I'd like to stress that we are all bio-individuals with different responses to food. This is why I do not go too deep with any single approach.

My *very* basic dietary advice in a nutshell:

- Seek a nutritional therapy practitioner[2] to determine your very personal bio-individual needs and establish a nutrition plan together.

---

2 https://nutritionaltherapy.com/provider-search/

- Value your meal time, eat in a relaxed state, and chew thoroughly.
- Increase your consumption of healthy fats and cut out highly processed (liquid-at-room-temperature) vegetable oils, Crisco, margarine, and any other oil that is chemically treated or heated. These oils have detrimental effects on our health.
- Cut out processed forms of carbohydrates such as breads, pasta, and treats, and increase your intake of all kinds of vegetables. Cut down on fructose-heavy fruits like apples, peaches, and oranges, and stick with berries, which are lower glycemic. Eat starchy vegetables such as sweet potatoes, yucca, and squashes after exercise to replace glycogen stores. ***If you lift heavy weights and do high intensity training,*** white rice (post-workout) is easily digested and can quickly refuel glycogen stores for better recovery.
- If there is one thing I have learned throughout my journey and past work with clients, it's that giving very *specific* nutrition advice to mass numbers is challenging. Again, we are all so different. Find what works best for your personal needs, which may change as you age. The key is finding what works and making the changes.

Here are a few books that represent some of the different approaches I recommend you explore to help you get started on your personal health journey:

- The Paleo Approach: Reverse Autoimmune Disease and Heal Your Body by Sarah Ballantyne[3]
- *Wired to Eat: Turn Off Cravings, Rewire Your Appetite for Weight Loss, and Determine the Foods That Work for You*, by Robb Wolf
- *It Starts With Food: Discover the Whole30 and Change Your Life in Unexpected Ways*
- *Real Food Keto: Applying Nutritional Therapy to Your Low-Carb, High-Fat Diet*
- Grain Brain by David Perlmutter
- Keto: The Complete Guide to Success on The Ketogenic Diet including Simplified Science and No-Cook Meal Plans by Maria Emmerich and Craig Emmerich
- The New Primal Blueprint by Mark Sisson (book and cookbook)
- Wild Fermentation by Sandor Ellix Katz and Sally Fallon Morell

3 This book is great for anyone struggling with autoimmune issues and has helped me tremendously.

Chapter 5

SUPPORTING PERIMENOPAUSE WITH SUPPLEMENTS

While honoring your moods and validating your feelings is of utmost importance, there are some supplements I highly recommend to help support more balanced moods and hormones throughout your cycle. These are just a few suggestions, and there are many more. I don't have all *your answers* because I don't know you. Once again, I recommend finding a doctor with a functional medicine approach to address the root cause of your hormonal imbalance. You may have excessive cortisol related to stress impacting your adrenals. Maybe you have an autoimmune-related thyroid issue. There are as many unique issues as there are women. This chapter is meant as an introduction to the topic of using supplements to support your health.

It's All Connected!

My go-to guru for all things female and hormonal is Dr. Jolene Brighten. Her work highlights how the hypothalamic pituitary and adrenal glands are all connected. Each system has a profound impact on the other. Dr. Brighten states that her patients tend to be focused on just one gland. For example, she often hears "It's just my thyroid" or "It's just my adrenals." However, it's never just one gland contributing to health symptoms. Each component of the endocrine system works together and communicates with the others. Dr. Brighten does thorough testing, digs deep, and helps her clients to find balance among these components. As Dr. Brighten puts it, "Your ovaries, adrenals, and thyroid are three legs on a stool. They are all the foundation to hormone balance."

Work with a professional to help you determine the root cause of what is happening in your body, and come up with a nutrition, lifestyle, and supplement plan that can help support your hormones and keep these body systems in balance.

Why am I even bringing up supplements? you might ask.

During Perimenopause, Progesterone Drops

There are many benefits to increasing our progesterone during early perimenopause, as progesterone typically drops before estrogen does. Progesterone is the feel good "chill" hormone. Progesterone stabilizes the lining of the uterus, helping us to conceive and maintain pregnancy. However, as progesterone begins to decline during perimenopause, so does our fertility. Progesterone benefits reach far beyond fertility.

Progesterone also:

- Helps with estrogen-related brain fog, and works synergistically with estrogen to produce the "feel good" neurotransmitters serotonin and dopamine (Barth, Villringer, and Sacher, 2015)
- Is considered to have a neuroprotective effect on the brain (Si, Li, Liu, Wang, Wei, Tian, Wang, and Liu, 2014)
- Provides cardiovascular benefits (Thomas and Pang, 2013)
- Protects against osteoporosis (Seifert-Klauss and Prior, 2010)
- Protects against some forms of hormone sensitive cancers, such as breast and ovarian (Ferretti, Felici, and Cognetti, 2007)

As progesterone declines, the severity of PMS may increase. Rather than focusing solely on decreasing excessive estrogens, we can also place some focus on naturally increasing our progesterone levels.

This can be done through:

- Managing stress (high stress levels affect progesterone)
- Getting adequate sleep at night
- Eating healthy fats (healthy fats help us to make healthy hormones)
- Using a bioidentical progesterone cream under the guidance of a healthcare professional. Bioidentical progesterone contains progesterone molecularly similar to the progesterone our body makes.
- Incorporating herbal adaptogens such as Ashwagandha, rhodiola, as well as B vitamins to help with decreasing cortisol, which affects our delicate hypothalamic-pituitary axis
- Getting adequate minerals such as magnesium and zinc, both of which are imperative for hundreds of enzymatic processes in the body

Supplements for Optimal Female Health

Although all women will eventually reach the end of their fertility life cycle, the journey does not have to be perilous. Here are a few key supplements I have found helpful with clients and from personal experience:

Ashwagandha

Ashwagandha is an Ayurvedic herbal adaptogen, which means it helps reduce cortisol (the stress hormone), therefore lowering stress levels. From experience, I argue that Ashwagandha works better than most other herbal adaptogens, in terms of stress response (Chandrasekhar, Kapoor, and Anishetty, 2012). I recommend taking it at night, as it can help with sleep as well.

**Please note: Ashwagandha is a nightshade, and therefore not recommended for people who are avoiding night-shades, such as people with certain autoimmune conditions who find they react to nightshades. A great alternative is rhodiola, another herbal adaptogen that can help with stress.*

CBD Oil

CBD (cannabidiol) is the non-psychoactive component to marijuana. CBD is known to possess many health benefits, one being that it helps with mood and anxiety (Blessing, Steenkamp, Manzanares, and Marmar, 2015). Many of us become more anxious during the luteal phase, and CBD helps with this anxiety. CBD is also anti-inflammatory in nature, which may help with spasm of the uterus, and menstrual cramping (Burstein, 2015).

Vitex

Vitex (Vitex agnus-castus) helps to regulate the endocrine system through targeting the hypothalamus-pituitary axis (Kashani, Hajaghaee, and Akhondzadeh, 2011). Vitex is the number one herb used in Europe for PMS-related symptoms such as mood swings, depression, and irritability. It does so through reducing the synthesis of follicle-stimulating hormones and estrogen, keeping everything more balanced.

Reishi Mushroom

Reishi mushroom ("the mushroom of eternal life") is an herbal adaptogen, which also possesses hepatoprotective (liver) benefits, therefore detoxing the liver. Reishi is amazing for insomnia, depression, and anxiety (Muhammad and Ali, 2017); it's high in antioxidants as well. Reishi is one of my favorite supplements. I love that it is a food-based supplement and very helpful for those struggling with autoimmunity, as it boosts immune health and fights cancer.

Topical Magnesium

Magnesium deficiency is a global epidemic. Magnesium chloride oil is by far my favorite product for managing PMS symptoms (I saved the best for last). Many women in our modern society are deficient in magnesium due to low dietary intake, depleted magnesium in our soil, modern stressors (stress depletes magnesium), consumption of carbonated beverages and coffee, and a nutrient-poor diet. Craving chocolate around PMS time? Chocolate is high in magnesium, and our requirements for magnesium increase as we approach menstruation. In fact, serum magnesium levels tend to be lower as we approach menstruation (Posaci, Erten, Uren, and Acar, 1994). Magnesium lowers anxiety and prevents insomnia. It also acts as a diuretic to help with swollen breasts and abdominal bloating.

For many of us struggling with digestive health issues, taking a supplement internally does not guarantee we are getting the nutrients from it. By using it topically, we are able to increase our magnesium levels and start to feel better fast! When I approach my monthly cycle, my sleep becomes more disrupted. Using magnesium lotion on my breasts, lower abdomen, and inner thighs right before bed helps me with breast tenderness, cramping, and sleep latency. As my period approaches and abdominal cramping become stronger, I find magnesium chloride bath soaks help tremendously to reduce body aches and cramping. I will dive deeper into magnesium in the sleep section. However, I feel it is one of the most important minerals for our health and well-being, and one most of us are deficient in.

Chapter 6

KEEPING SEXUALITY ALIVE AS WE AGE

We are sexual beings. Sexual energy is life force. It's our core energy, our vibrancy, our passion. However, when it comes to females and aging, there are so many deep-seated beliefs surrounding our sexuality that we just "don't go there.“ We want to have more sex and better sex. We want to feel alive in our sexuality, yet many of us feel sexually repressed or held back. What are some of the root issues holding us back?

This bears repeating: sexual energy is our core life force. It drives so much of our passion and spreads to all areas of our life. It adds to our zest for life, our creativity, our passions. Yet many women are unaware that they *are* sexual beings or possess this amazing core energy within ourselves.

There are so many cultural messages thrown at women surrounding our sexuality. We've been taught that being sexual equals being promiscuous or bad or wrong. We have deeply held psychological beliefs surrounding our sexuality based upon how we have been conditioned. Society bombards us with messages about our sexuality, including messages about violence, harassment, the government trying to take a role in our personal sexual decisions, sex addiction, pornography, youth, body image, and so much more. Many of us have experienced harassment or abuse and associate our sexuality with shame. All of these messages and experiences play a role in shaping our core sexual beliefs, and they affect our ability to embrace a positive sexual identity.

What are your core beliefs surrounding sexuality? What comes up for you? Many women feel a great deal of guilt and shame surrounding sexuality. Our culture wants women to be sexual but not too sexual. Our very skewed version of what is considered "sexy" is built and perpetuated by the media.

Cultivating the Creative Force of Sexuality

I spoke with the amazing Bridget Finn, Ph.D. Finn is the founder and president of The Capital Region Center for Sexual Health, a sex therapist, and a researcher with over thirty years of experience. We had an amazing conversation surrounding sexuality and the older female.

As we age, many of us believe our sexuality ends. Sex is marketed toward the young and the beautiful. According to Finn:

> *When you think about perimenopause, what does the culture tell us? What are we being sold? What are we buying? We are buying into: I'm old, I'm dry, I'm going to gain weight, it's over.* (Bridget Finn, pers. comm.)

Well, that's a load of bull! As we age, our sexuality or life energy becomes even more intense and amazing. However, we have to nurture and expand it. We have to let go of any shame we have created around our sexual identity over the years. This isn't an overnight process, and it takes some personal reflection and work.

Finn suggests that when women hit a certain age, typically mid-forties and into our fifties, we start to feel invisible to men. We may stop turning heads. We feel no one really sees us anymore; therefore, we feed into this invisibility and often stop investing in ourselves and our sexuality. Finn states, "Perhaps there is an invisibility to men, but there is not an invisibility to ourselves, and the other people in our lives." Women at this stage in life have a vibrancy about them. We're alive in ways we don't realize, and when we take the time to nurture this vibrancy, we create amazing sexual energy beyond our wildest imagination.

We think we lose our libido as we age. We believe our sexual time is over and our sexuality ends with menopause. What we don't realize is that our libido needs to be nurtured to be kept alive, and that our libido is our creativity, our passion, our driving force. We have to make a conscious effort to nurture our libido. It needs to be fed, or it starves. Dr. Finn suggests that your libido needs to be inspired: "Our sexuality needs to be put on the front burner, on a low boil, all the time." It is not something that you just let sit and then wonder why it dies.

> *My uncle use to have this car that he would leave out in the winter for months and never turn it on. Then in the spring, he would struggle with getting it to start. As women we are taught that our sexual activity depends upon another person. We think that someone needs to come along and just make it happen for us. However, our libido is our job. It's our mojo, our energy. We are responsible for turning the engine on frequently and firing it up.* (Bridget Finn, pers. comm.)

According to Finn, the number one issue holding women back is that they aren't giving themselves permission to be sexual beings. Do you masturbate?

Do you feel like you need to have permission to pleasure yourself? Do you believe self-pleasure is something dirty, wrong, or bad because of how you were conditioned growing up? In the same way that muscle can atrophy if we neglect proper physical exercise, vaginal tissue can atrophy, thinning and drying as we age. Sexual pleasure, whether it be self-pleasure or pleasure from a partner, keeps the vagina full of blood, moisturized, and vibrant. ***Masturbation is part of our self-care***, yet so many of us do not give ourselves permission. The orgasm releases stress and increases feel good chemicals to the brain, such as dopamine and serotonin. According to Finn, for most women, their vagina is foreign. We have little to no body awareness in that entire area. No blood flow. No stimulation. No feeling. We just let it die.

Sexual energy is not stagnant. Many Americans are living single now. The demographic has shifted. Just because you are single doesn't mean you are not a sexual being.

> *When it comes to somebody coming in for therapy, stating they are in peri-menopause and no longer have a libido, there's a whole lot that isn't happening that needs to get that libido fired up. I always ask them, are you feeling joy in your life? Are you feeling alive? Are you tapping into your creativity? Are you in a relationship that's inspiring you? That's*

> *compelling you? Is it additive, not just neutral, but is it bringing joy to you?* (Bridget Finn, pers. comm.)

The issue is that we are not nurturing, renewing, expanding, rejuvenating, redetermining, and re-exploring. Finn concludes, "With perimenopause, my message to women is that you cannot be living your life the way you were twenty years ago" (Bridget Finn, pers. comm.).

Evolving Sexuality

According to Finn, "Everything has changed. People change. Jobs change. Landscapes changed. Why on earth would our sexuality remain the same? People have a *static* perspective of sexuality and relationships" (Bridget Finn, pers. comm.). As we grow and change, so does our sexuality, and so do our desires. Why are we remaining stagnant? Just because our sexuality changes as we age, it doesn't mean it ends. We just have to make our sexuality a priority. The result? Other areas of our life begin to flourish as well.

Are you married or in a monogamous relationship? Monogamy does not have to be monotonous. We make it that way because we stop doing the hard work. Couples get comfortable in the day-to-day monotony. They get set in their ways. Then it becomes scary to reinvent and reinvigorate ourselves. Finn suggests, "If we were as unconscious in our jobs as we are in our relationships, we would be fired" (Bridget Finn, pers. comm.). We have sex in the same room, and in the same way, and at the same time. Do you eat boiled chicken for every meal, every day? People get bored. We need adventure.

We have to be willing to be adventurous as a sexual couple to feel alive inside. Sexual energy is vibrancy. The biggest lie we feed ourselves is that sex is a chore. Our sexual energy is not the same energy we use to get through the day, to take care of the kiddos, yet we compartmentalize it right there with the grocery list and the mortgage payment. Our sexuality is not part of our to-do list, yet we schedule it in as if it were. Having sex becomes yet another task that needs to be accomplished and checked off the list. How is that fulfilling?

There are many factors we need to consider in order to maintain our libido as we age. Movement is huge. We need to move our bodies, which helps to keep our energy flowing and not stagnant. Nutrition, grounding (skin-to-earth contact), sunlight, and prayer/meditation are also very important. All of these are important for all aspects of our life as we age. However, we need to let go of the idea that after menopause we are no longer sexual beings. This is such a big lie. Please don't succumb to this. Sexual contact with yourself or a partner helps to release stress and correlates with better health as we age.

We need to feel alive. We need this life force energy because it expands into all that we do. However, one of the biggest factors here is our relationships. **Our relationships become our essence, and if our essence is stale and boring, so is our sexuality.** It feels safe and comfortable for us to become stagnant in our sexual relationships. We don't want to do the hard work to maintain it. We think it should just happen for us, and if it doesn't, we just don't have it anymore. We have to be active participants in our sexuality. *Having a good sexual relationship is a lifestyle choice, not something that just happens with chemistry.* The chemistry helps early on when someone in our life is new. However, we have to make that lifestyle choice to nurture our sexuality, to leave the state of comfort and ease, and to do the hard work.

Research shows sexual expression has positive effects on decreased mortality, lower frequency of fatal coronary events, and decreased risk of breast cancer in men and women. Sexual expression also increases general well-being, pain management, and general quality of life. We should not assume that as we age we can no longer enjoy great sex and experience powerful sexual energy. Being able to openly express our sexuality is one of the most exciting opportunities we have as we age! We just need to let go of societal and cultural expectations surrounding sexuality. We must allow ourselves to flourish as natural sexual beings!

What can we do to bring out our sexual energy?

Finn suggests we can't just "wait until we might feel something." We have to communicate with our partner and allow ourselves to be vulnerable, open, and honest. A spark will not just come out of nowhere, unless our relationship is very new. Love is work. Sex is a gift. Do the hard stuff. Talk openly and honestly about your emotional and sexual needs. It's uncomfortable and unconventional, but it's the only way to truly allow for your sexual needs to be met. Opening up to our partner, being vulnerable, and expressing our needs and desires are all extremely important for our sexual health, as well as our emotional, physical, and spiritual health.

Touch yourself. Masturbate. Get familiar with your body. Use a mirror and get to know your vagina on a personal level. Don't be ashamed of vibrators. It's okay to feel good. There is nothing bad or wrong about being a sexual being. Embrace your sexuality and work through any sexual blocks you may be holding due to past experiences and limiting beliefs stemming all the way back to childhood. Although you may carry some deep-seated shame surrounding your sexuality, understand that sexuality does not equal shame. Work through and let go of false beliefs surrounding your sexuality. Talk it through with a therapist if need be. You are deserving of a healthy and vibrant sexual life well into old age.

Chapter 7
GROUNDING/EARTHING

Our modern lifestyle has us pretty much cooped up indoors, sitting throughout most of the day. We are more disconnected from our planet than ever before. We wear thick, factory-made rubber soled shoes (which we start wearing as infants), we have hard floors and desks. We are keeping our body off the earth, when touching the earth has absolutely amazing health benefits.

Earthing or *grounding* reconnects us with our natural environment through a transfer of electrons from the earth into our physical body. The earth's surface possesses a limitless and continuously renewed supply of electrons (Chevalier, Sinatra, Oschman, Sokal, and Sokal, 2012). Does this all seem too woo-woo for you? Research is proving that grounding is legit.

Earthing possesses amazing health benefits, and it's free! Connecting with the earth decreases feelings of depression and anxiety; it decreases pain and improves immune health, cardiovascular health, and sleep (Oschman, Chevalier, and Brown, 2015). Earthing shifts the body from a sympathetic (fight or flight) to a parasympathetic (relaxed) state (Chevalier, et al., 2012). The only requirement? Go outside and walk barefoot.

Earthing also helps with getting adequate sleep. Many people have a difficult time falling asleep and staying asleep, and modern stress is a huge contributor to the problem. The sleep medication industry makes a fortune in sleep aids. The earth's negative electrons help to create an internal rhythm within our body, which in turn helps to set our circadian rhythm, or sleep cycle, telling our body when to appropriately secrete specific hormones like cortisol and melatonin (Oschman, 2008).

In one study, measurable improvements in diurnal cortisol profiles were observed with grounding, with cortisol levels significantly reduced during nighttime sleep (Ghaly and Teplitz, 2004). Grounding during sleep not only reduced cortisol, but also re-synchronized the participant's hormone secretions to align with a more natural twenty-four-hour circadian rhythm. The subjects also reported reduced pain and stress!

One great way to ground at night, is to use grounding mats or sheets with your bed. The earth has a slightly negative charge, and grounding mats absorb this charge from the earth, and allow it to be absorbed into the body through our feet. Grounding mats or sheets allow for the electrons in the earth to be absorbed into your tissue, as if you were standing directly on the earth.

Less cortisol = better sleep = better overall mood.

The earth's electrons have also been shown to neutralize free radicals and boost the health of our immune system. Our ancestors not only walked barefoot or wore animal skins (through which the earth's electrons are absorbed), oftentimes they slept with their body directly on the earth. This contact with the earth while sleeping neutralizes free radicals and stabilizes all of our organs, tissues, and cells.

Earthing also reduces inflammation in the body (Oschman, 2007). These anti-inflammatory effects are due to negatively charged antioxidant electrons from the earth entering the body and neutralizing positively charged free radicals, thereby reducing overall inflammation in the body. This is great news for people struggling with modern inflammatory conditions such as autoimmune disorders. Earthing also accelerated the immune response to vaccinations.

Earthing the body might be the primary modulator of the endocrine and nervous system (Sokal and Sokal, 2011). In a double-blind pilot study, a biofeedback system recorded the electrophysiological and physiological parameters of thirty healthy control subjects (Chevalier, et al., 2012). Upon earthing, about half of the subjects showed an abrupt change in EEG. Earthing changed the electrophysiological properties of the participants' brains and musculature for the better. There were overall reductions in stress and tension, and a shift in the autonomic nervous system immediately upon earthing. Grounding also improved heart rate variability, supporting cardiovascular health, improving all the way to the end of a forty-minute grounding period (Chevalier and Sinatra, 2011). This suggests that earthing has a greater heart rate variability benefit with increased time.

In patients who experience anxiety, emotional stress, panic, fear, and/or symptoms of autonomic dystonia, including headaches, cardiac palpitations, and dizziness, grounding could be a very realistic therapy. These patients may see positive effects most likely within twenty to thirty minutes and in almost all cases in forty minutes. Depression and anxiety symptoms such as panic, sadness, hostility, etc. all affect heart rate variability, illustrated in the reality that depression and anxiety are linked to cardiovascular disease. Earthing helps to switch the body into a parasympathetic or relaxed state, balancing the autonomic nervous system, thus decreasing depression, further decreasing risks of cardiovascular events for depressed patients with cardiovascular disease.

Earthing showed significant changes in minerals and electrolytes in blood serum—in just one night! The observed reductions in calcium and phosphorus were directly related to osteoporosis. A single night of grounding can help reduce some primary indicators for osteoporosis (Chevalier, et al., 2012).

Earthing also shows promising help for thyroid function (Ober, Sinatra, and Zucker, 2010)! One night of grounding produces a significant decrease in thyroid-stimulating hormones. Many individuals taking thyroid medication found that grounding with medication actually increased hyperthyroid symptoms, thus needing to work with their doctor and adjust their medication downward. The thyroid is the master gland affecting all physiological processes in the body. Earthing just may be the primary modulator for our endocrine health!

In a pilot study, earthing decreased delayed muscle soreness (DOMS) in participants (Brown, Chevalier, and Hill, 2010). In another study, healthy men ages 20–23 were put through a similar routine of toe raises while carrying on their shoulders a barbell equal to one-third of their body weight (Chevalier, et al., 2012). Researchers grounded half the participants and tested their blood chemistry and pain levels. The researchers concluded that grounding the body to the earth alters measures of immune system activity and pain. The ungrounded participants experienced a strong increase in white blood cells (associated with decreased inflammatory response) at the stage when DOMS is known to reach its peak and greater perception of pain. The grounded men, however, had only a slight decrease in white blood cells, indicating scant inflammation, and a shorter recovery time. Therefore, simply by connecting with the earth, we can recover more quickly from our body's innate response to muscle trauma!

Getting outside and connecting with the earth for as little as a half hour per day can have a significant positive impact on our overall physical and mental health! Plus, it doesn't cost anything. Granted it is more difficult to get outside and ground in the colder months, especially for those living in colder climates. However, there are special conductive shoes that can be worn outside. Unlike synthetic factory-made shoes, animal skin moccasins, as our ancestors wore, are also conductive to the earth's electrons. So get outside, play outside, walk barefoot, work outside when you can, and sleep on the earth. The more you can, the better you will feel. Cheers to grounding/earthing and good health!

Chapter 8

MAKING TIME FOR MOVEMENT AND PLAY

Prolonged sitting has been associated with cancer, heart disease, type 2 diabetes, muscular issues, and increased risk of depression ("Ways Sitting Is Shortening Your Life", 2015). As we age, it is imperative that we move our bodies throughout the day. Getting movement throughout the day, is more important than scheduling one intense exercise session. If you have a sedentary job, get up and walk, or stretch frequently. Taking time each day to move our bodies is necessary for both our mental and physical health.

Many of us are attached to the idea that we need to do intense physical exercise, like strength training at the gym, distance running, or heavy lifting. Movement does not have to be intense physical exercise in order for you to reap the benefits. In fact, many of us are overtraining, and this puts the body into an inflamed state and can make us feel worse. Movement is cumulative throughout the day. Every half hour, we should get up and move our body.

Many yogis attest to the benefits of being inverted, or upside down. Being upside down is an amazing way to reinvigorate ourselves and get blood flowing to the brain! It has been praised for providing better circulation, increased energy, lymphatic drainage, and a host of other benefits. If you can't do a handstand or headstand (I'm one of those who cannot quite do that yet), simply getting in downward-facing dog pose and peddling out the feet is an amazing way to get mostly inverted and get that blood flow to the brain.

What about cardio and strength training? I'm very big on *functional movement.* Functional movements involve movement that incorporates many large muscles, rather than isolating specific muscles. Functional movement utilizes the core stabilizers and all different planes of movement. In our culture, we love to isolate things. There is this concept when it comes to health that is important to remember: Our body systems are *synergistic.* All our muscles, joints, and ligaments, work together. Western doctors treat individual symptoms rather than looking at the whole picture. We love to separate and isolate our muscles when we lift weights, focusing on just one or two muscle groups per session. In a sense, we are micromanaging our body. Movement can be exciting, fun, and all-encompassing of the entire body. You don't have to dread leg day at the gym any longer.

Many of us shy away from physical activity based solely upon years of conditioning. We believe exercise is something demanded of us, something that is not fun, and something that we often associate with dread. We call it *fitness*. And *exercise*. And *training*.

> *Functional movement should translate into every context and purpose, including sports playing, gardening, running after and picking up children, and even walking through the shopping mall.* (Georges Dagher, 2017)

Let's change this paradigm and simply call it *movement*.

Movement in Your Forties

Movement in our forties is important because it releases growth hormones, which help to keep us young and active. Sarcopenia is an alteration in structure, biochemistry, and molecular function of muscles associated with aging. Sarcopenia creates frailty, poor quality of life, and an early death. We want to feel good in our middle age. We want quality of life over longevity. Many factors lead to loss of strength, but the primary causes are oxidative stress, hormonal changes, reduced physical activity, insulin resistance, and nutritional deficiencies. The best way to counteract sarcopenia as we age is through movement. The signaling pathways in our muscles are modulated through movement. We need to move our bodies. *Movement is absolutely necessary to a woman's ability to survive and thrive.*

Movement is therapeutic for memory and brain function, and it releases hormones that help to keep us vibrant and feeling good (Diederich, Bastl, Wersching, Teuber, Strecker, Schmidt, Minnerup, and Schabitz, 2017; Ignacio, Silvestre, Albuquerque, Andrade, Carvalho, Castro, 2015)! CrossFit is an excellent choice for women seeking regular movement. Although there are poor-quality places that can give CrossFit a bad name, I recommend finding a facility that places an emphasis on mobility as part of the training and employs coaches who are strict about correct form. Sometimes it takes trial and error to find a quality place, but CrossFit is a great option for many people, so don't be afraid to try. I also realize CrossFit might not be a great fit for everyone. I typically don't go to CrossFit more than a few times a week (usually three to four), as I struggle with autoimmune issues. Any over-stress to the body, even good stress, can cause an autoimmune flare-up for me. My goal is to keep my body as uninflamed as possible. This requires

I let go of my ego sometimes and take full rest days, or days where walking my dog is my most strenuous form of movement.

On days I do not go to CrossFit, I incorporate yoga, stretching, walking my dog, biking, wrestling with my boys, hiking, and sex. Yes, even sex is movement! These are all beneficial movements that utilize the body.

With this said, I believe it is very important for women to lift heavy things, at least two to three times a week. We do lose muscle tissue as we get older, and it's important to maintain our strength. If you do not have access to equipment or can't allocate funds to a gym membership for lifting weights, you can still use your own body for resistance training. A recent study actually showed that high repetition, low-load exercise (such as push-ups, lunges, wall squats, sit-ups, etc.) produced significantly greater increases in growth hormone (Fink, Kikuchi, and Nakazato, 2016). Second, there were long-term extra gains in the muscle cross-sectional areas and muscle thickness in the group that did the low-load, high-rep training. What this means for us is that you don't even need a gym. Just a section of floor and maybe a pull-up bar. There are countless videos out there with various routines you can follow.

Get Squatting!

There is one movement I think everyone should work on *daily,* and that is the deep squat! Georges Dagher, DC, writes that deep squatting is the "toothbrush to our joints" helping to align everything (2017). Squatting helps to align the shoulders, spine, knees, hips, and ankles, and isn't just for CrossFitters. Squatting helps with mobility, stability, strength, balance, and coordination, at every age and every level.

According to Dagher:

> *When discussing movement and spine health, there's a Chinese proverb that comes to mind: "You are as old as your spine."*
>
> *This proverb resonates with me on multiple levels:*
>
> *As a student, when I sat for long period of time, my back would ache.*
>
> *As an athlete, if I sat on the bench for a long time, my back would feel stiff.*
>
> *As driver, when I'm sitting for long period of time in traffic, I feel stuck, stiff, and achy.*
>
> *As I watch my loved ones age, my uncles, parents, grandparents, I can visually observe stiffness as it develops within them.*

In one of my publications discussing joint health and low back pain, I touched on a popular contemporary colloquialism: "sitting is the new smoking." My challenge to the reader was that if indeed sitting is the new smoking, then standing is similar to the Nicotine patch, a short upright static solution that eventually, if maintained beyond the body's capacity, is a common provocative source of lower back pain.

What does this all mean? If movement is indeed the most potent natural anti-inflammatory prescription, then the effects "hinge" on our ability to move! Remaining in any static position directly affects our movement, not only during that period but beyond, leading to stiffness. This makes movement significantly more difficult when we finally decide to move.

From a longevity standpoint, the solution would be to simply move. The barrier to entry is low, as the sole prerequisite would be to have a body capable of movement, be it walking, squatting, balancing, a mixture of these movements and others, etc. Once you begin to move, you can then dive deeper into the areas of your body that need more attention than others. Maybe your back feels stiff and achy, so those cat-camel exercises your doctor or trainer told you to do have a purpose. Maybe you realize one of your

> *hips is tight or stiff, and that hip opener/stretch now makes sense.*
>
> *In order to take advantage of movement, we need to move well and for a sustained period of time. Movement is advantageous for our joints and muscles and encourages them to work with us instead of against us: "if we are stiff and tight when we move, we won't move. If we feel great when we move, we will move more.* (pers. comm.)

Georges suggests the best bodyweight movement to work on daily is the deep squat. You ever notice how toddlers naturally squat so easily? It's a functional movement that offers so many amazing benefits.

The bodyweight deep squat.

Dagher suggests:

> *The squat is a form of communication between the squatter and their physical or social environment. The ability to descend into the deep squat requires a healthy mix of joint mobility, stability, strength, and coordination. Priming the body for the deep squat, and utilizing it as much as possible, creates an opportunity for improved function and overall mobility. In my opinion, the deep squat can serve as a daily movement ritual or test that gives you information about your body. Whether you're a*

> *powerlifter, weightlifter, CrossFitter, weekend warrior, or a parent, the ability to squat directly impacts your life, lifestyle, social interaction, and health. Picking up a barbell, baby, or a bag of groceries off the floor is all founded on that hinge, which is engraved in the deep squat.* (pers. comm.)

Practice getting deeper and deeper into the squat each time, keeping your weight in your heels, abdomen tight, and your chest up. You can stick your arms out in front of you for balance. Hold for five to ten seconds and repeat. Work your way up to a twenty-second hold and three sets of five throughout the day. You can also challenge yourself and add dumbbells or work on pistols, squatting with one leg extended forward.

I asked Stephanie Gaudreau of Stupid Easy Paleo and author of The Paleo Athlete what her favorite functional movement was, and Steph said:

> *I really love the goblet squat as an introduction to functional movement. As a society we spend so much time sitting at or above parallel. Getting down into a deep squat with a little bit of weight out front is a great way to establish what your mobility and stability are like before you proceed with heavier squat variations or barbell squats.* (pers. comm.)

What about Playing?

Man only plays when he is in the fullest sense of the word a human being, and he is only fully a human being when he plays.
– Friedrich Schiller

Wait what? I'm an adult. Why are we going there?

We have also lost the art of playing and being playful. As adults, we still need to play! We get so wrapped up in the responsibilities of daily life that we forget just how to truly *live* at times. Those childhood carefree moments of letting go and playing become fleeting. Why not welcome more of this into our lives as a way to offset the (gazillion) modern stressors we face?

Play is just as imperative for adults as it is for children. However, culturally it's seen as unnecessary, and frivolous. We just forget because we're trying so hard to be an adult. This doesn't mean we don't truly need play. Neglecting playfulness can lead us to adopt maladaptive behaviors in order to cope with life stressors.

Don Miguel Ruiz writes:

> *The happiest moments in our lives are when we are playing just like children, we are singing and dancing, when we are exploring and creating just for fun. It is wonderful when we behave like a*

> *child because this is the normal human tendency. As children, we are innocent, and it is natural for us to express love. But what has happened to us? What has happened to the whole world?* (Ruiz, 2011)

Many of us still hold onto that desire to play, yet we stifle it because of adult expectations. We get so wrapped up in the confines of our daily structures and routines that play becomes something very foreign to us. This makes it more difficult for us to feel relaxed, let loose, and just be silly. We tend to want to structure and schedule everything, rather than letting go and just being in the moment.

Here are some amazing benefits to unstructured play:

Unstructured play reduces stress and improves stress response.

Researchers have found that people who are playful reported lower levels of perceived stress than less playful people and had better strategies in place for coping with stressful situations. The playful people were less likely to engage in negative, avoidant, and escaping behaviors.

Playing = Less stress = lower cortisol = better sleep = better hormones = better mood

Play reduces symptoms of depression.

According to Dr. Stuart Brown, founder and president of the National Institute for Play and author of Play: How it Shapes the Brain, Opens the Imagination and Invigorates the Soul, adults who exhibit playfulness possess more positive indicators of psychological and physical well-being and are more satisfied with their life.

Play contributes to healthy hormones.

According Darryl Edwards, author of Animal Moves:

> *Play invokes the feel good hormones – endorphins, dopamine, and serotonin - the key to some incredible mental health benefits, including improved mood, reduced stress and anxiety, greater happiness and a feeling of being more alive. These are easily generated through active play, especially when involving other individuals which can introduce oxytocin release too.* (2016)

Most of us believe play is only for children. Culturally we tend to see play as unproductive, and we like to "hustle" and stay busy, even though a great deal of our busyness is not really productive. However, we still require playfulness, even as adults. This desire does not go away; we just stifle it. It's part of our human design. When we honor this, we tend to be healthier and less violent. This doesn't mean you are not a responsible person or a good parent for letting loose and playing. You are actually much less agitated when you play, and you're probably a better parent.

Researchers tested playfulness with strength of character in adults. Single strengths of creativity, zest, and hope were strongly related to playfulness. "Fun" people were most strongly related to having emotional strength, and intellectual strength was strongly associated with all variables of playfulness.

Play helps children learn how to respond to situations they encounter and strengthens their emotional health. This is true for adults too, at a different level. If you have old emotional wounds that never quite healed, playing can help bring feelings up gently and release them in a fun and loving way.

Playing is a great relationship tool. It can really strengthen a bond, bring couples closer, and allow them to work through and let go of old thought patterns. This can truly strengthen our adult relationships and friendships.

In his book Healing the Child Within, Charles Whitfield discusses how we have an inner child, or true self, yet we stifle and hide this fun and playful part of ourselves from the world. He refers to enjoyment and fun as an altered state of consciousness, and he believes we need to experience these altered states from time to time.

Actually we seem to have an innate—even biological need—to periodically alter our conscious state, whether it be by daydreaming, laughing, playing sports, concentrating on a project, or sleeping. (2015)

Whitfield suggests we need to have fun. Go figure!

Playfulness is always there, available inside us, however, we have to make a conscious effort to let go and bring the joy out. Here are some fun ideas to try:

- Play an adult game of tag, Duck–Duck Goose, Simon Says, or Red Rover.
- Dance party! (Need I say more?)
- Wrestle in the grass, or on the beach (with your spouse, significant other, kids, dog, or friends).
- When you take your kids sledding, hop in a sled too! Or go sledding without kids.
- Use your imagination and pretend.
- Role-play and fantasy during sex is actually a form of free play.
- Skip, hop, run, leap, jump rope.
- Jump waves in the ocean.
- Tell "stupid" jokes.

In our technological age, it's important that we take time out of our day (even just a few minutes) to do something silly, fun, and unstructured. The benefits to our physical and emotional health are irreplaceable. We get so stuck in our structured ways, whereas play has no expected outcome, time line, or expectations. This allows for us to fully immerse ourselves in the moment and release the buildup of stress that develops over time!

Let go, and play!

Chapter 9

GETTING ADEQUATE SLEEP

Sleep? What's that? It's something that *most* of us are not getting enough of. We have a lot of societal pressure on us to stay up late and to sleep in. I have been referred to as a "little old lady" because I go to bed sometimes as early as 8:30 p.m., and I typically wake around 5 a.m. I have a strong awareness of my internal rhythm, and my body literally turns off after 8 p.m. However, I am my best, sharpest, most clear self early in the morning. This is *my* internal clock. I feel it so strongly that if I need to catch a flight or wake up early, I will instinctually wake up one minute before my alarm goes off, every single time. We all have a circadian rhythm, but many of us just don't have that deep of an awareness because we are so distracted by life.

Recent research by the National Center for Health Statistics(1) showed that one-third of women in their forties and fifties are chronically sleep deprived. In fact, "perimenopausal women were more likely than premenopausal and postmenopausal women to sleep less than 7 hours" (Vahratian, 2017). Perimenopausal women are having difficulty falling asleep and staying asleep. Lack of quality sleep impacts all areas of our health and well-being, yet it tends to be the last thing we address!

We face pressure at work, pressure with children and sports, pressure with fitting in our movement, all the other challenges life throws at us—and, in order to cope, one of the first things we tend to do away with is getting adequate sleep. We lie in bed at night, and our heads are just reeling with things we want to remember. Thinking about checklists. Thinking about the person you forgot to respond to earlier. Thinking about how horrible you are that you didn't smile enough when your son showed you his picture. Everything builds up during the day like a gigantic volcano, making it laughable when "sleep experts" give us tips on how to wind down at night. In the past I believed there was something seriously wrong with me because trying out those sleep tips just increased my anxiety surrounding sleep. However, sleep.is.life. I cannot stress this enough. So how can we fix this?

And it's not just our mental and emotional health that are affected by lack of sleep. Our physical health suffers greatly when we don't prioritize rest. According to an article in the International Journal of Genomics, "Disruptions of the circadian rhythms in shift workers are known risk factors for psychiatric disorders, gastrointestinal alterations, sleep and cognitive impairments, and breast cancer" (Kahn, 2018).

Let's look at the sleep patterns of a caveman, without electricity. Circadian rhythms, or our internal twenty-four-hour clock are dependent upon the season and the sun. Ancient humans were not staring at blue lights right before bed or working in buildings with artificial lights beaming down on them all day long. The body biologically followed the rhythm of the sun and the seasons. Sleep-wake cycles were guided by that first light kissing their skin in the morning.

This natural rhythm is part of our inherent biology, down to the cellular level. Our trillions of microbes in our microbiome both follow and are influenced by our circadian rhythm. Therefore, our sleep cycle plays a much more critical role in our health than we realized. The composition and structure of our microbiome are regulated by our own circadian rhythm. Our "master" clock is regulated by pacemaker neurons that oscillate in our brain, but also in *all* of our cells, and hormone receptors. We now know that this sleep-wake cycle controls our metabolism down to the cellular level. Down to our genetic expression.

Sleep loss has been associated with cancer, heart disease, Alzheimer's, weight loss resistance, and decreased cognitive performance—just to name a few. A new study showed that those people experiencing high levels of stress and sleep loss had much higher cognitive impairment and memory loss and decreased attention span. Most of us are experiencing moderate to high stress, just through our adult responsibilities and relationships.

Why Sleep Matters

What does this means for us? Why does it matter in the discussion of perimenopause? Sleep needs to be one of our top priorities—it's possibly the most important thing to prioritize. Yet for many of us, sleep is the first thing to go on the back burner. Getting adequate sleep is imperative for everything we've talked about so far. It's essential for growth hormone release and muscle repair. Sleep is also central to our hormonal health, mood, energy, weight, mental health, and cognition.

We are not placing a strong enough emphasis on getting adequate sleep. We are staying up late to watch our favorite shows. We are staring at screens before bed, scrolling through social media, and reading our Kindle books, which affects our ability to reach deep restorative sleep. We are taking over-the-counter and prescription medications to help us fall asleep and stay asleep. We have developed such an anxiety and pressure surrounding sleep that it just does not come naturally anymore. We are essentially a bunch of insomniacs running throughout the day in fight or flight. This has a profound effect on our moods, hormones, metabolism, relationships, sexuality, and overall health.

Throughout my twenties and early thirties, I struggled with severe anxiety surrounding sleep. I was so tired of "sleep experts" listing ways to get a good night's sleep, but none of it worked for me. Deep breathing didn't work. Meditation didn't work. Relaxing routines became anxiety-provoking routines because I believed they weren't going to work for me—and they didn't. Sleep became a battleground, and this impacted all aspects of my life, my marriage, my mental health, and my hormones. Meditation works great for many people, but it never worked for me.

What worked for me? I've literally run the gauntlet when it comes to sleep, and here are the top approaches that have helped me—and my clients—with both falling asleep and staying asleep. You may find other things work better for you. However, following these steps has been life-changing for me, and I have been sleeping beautifully since following this routine.

Getting morning sunlight on our skin is one of the most important ways to get good sleep at night. We literally have photoreceptors all over our body. Our skin takes in this sunlight and helps produce melatonin, a hormone that improves our ability to fall asleep (sleep latency) and stay asleep at night. When we are exposed to dim or artificial lights in the morning, we do not get the signals to produce sufficient melatonin in the evening (Kozaki, Toda, Noguchi, and Yasukouchi, 2011). Sunlight, especially first light of the morning, corresponds to better sleep at night. This is especially true in climates where it gets very cold, and we aren't outside as much. It's imperative in the winter to bundle up and get outside first thing in the morning, even if only for twenty minutes. I can't stress enough how much this morning light sets the tone for sleep at night!

Why We Can't Just Rely on Melatonin

The problem with taking melatonin at night? Melatonin is not an herbal supplement. It's actually a strong hormone, that regulates our body's internal clock. It tells our brain, "Time to go night–night." It does not contain any secret ingredient that helps you with decreasing the time it takes for your body to fall asleep. It's great to take when you are traveling and switching time zones (to help with resetting your rhythm to a new time zone). However, taken long term, melatonin alters hormones and may potentially numb hormone receptors. This is not something we really want from a sleep aid. I personally do not recommend melatonin for long-term use.

Magnesium is our best friend when it comes to sleep. According to Carolyn Dean MD, author of The Magnesium Miracle, most of us are deficient in magnesium. Due to modern farming practices, our soils are depleted of this essential mineral. Each time we are stressed (any kind, mental or physical) our body utilizes our stored magnesium. Magnesium supports over 400 enzymatic processes in our body. Dean attributes a myriad of psychological problems to magnesium deficiency. What I'm saying here as briefly as possible is that magnesium is pretty darn important, which is why I talk about it a few times in this book.

Magnesium is known as the calming mineral, aiding the brain in regulating excessive cortisol related to stress. Magnesium helps reduce the release of adrenocorticotropic hormone (ACTH), and it has a direct impact on the function of the transport of protein p-glycoprotein, which can influence the access of corticosteroids to the brain. All of these systems are involved in the pathophysiology of stress. Therefore, not only does magnesium help to relax tense/tight muscles, it also helps to relieve stress and anxiety we may feel before bed (when the infamous monkey brain starts going). There are many forms of magnesium, some are more easily digested and assimilated than others.

Here are my favorite *forms* of magnesium, and I personally recommend *both forms* every single night:

Topical Magnesium

One may assume a topical application doesn't enter the bloodstream. However, researchers are finding that topical applications do help raise our intracellular magnesium levels. Plus, if you can get your partner to massage it on, you also get a relaxing massage along with the benefits of magnesium. With some of the oil spray, you may find a slight tingling sensation, burning, or itching. Many people find that this goes away after a few uses. How much do I recommend? I typically use about five to ten pumps/sprays. I also lift heavy weights, which depletes magnesium (as does stress). Personally, I don't believe we can use too much topical magnesium. However, I always recommend consulting with your functional medicine practitioner on dosing.

Magnesium glycinate

There are many forms of ingestible magnesium, and you can find what works best for you. My favorite form is magnesium glycinate (400mg) because it is bound with glycine, making it easier for your body to digest and utilize the magnesium. Other forms of magnesium, such as magnesium citrate may make some people feel bloated or nauseated. However, other people do great with those forms. The key is finding a form that is right for *you.* I recommend taking 400mg every night with the topical magnesium.

Other Tips for Maximizing Sleep

Blue light–blocking glasses do just what it sounds like: they block blue light. What is blue light? Blue light is part of the light spectrum that has a very short wavelength and produces a high amount of energy. Blue light can come from the sun, light bulbs, televisions, cell phones, laptops, iPads, and reading tablets ("Shine the Light on Blue Light", n.d.).

Blue light from the sun peaks during the daytime. Our ancestors would be in sync with the sun and go to sleep when the sun sets. However, we are exposed to artificial lighting all day long and into the evening. We may think this isn't really doing anything, but it's doing a whole lot! Exposure to blue light before bed disrupts our circadian rhythm and can make it difficult for us to fall asleep and stay asleep, through inhibiting that melatonin that we so beautifully stepped outside in the morning to create. Being on a device just before bedtime induces circadian phase delay and melatonin suppression, alters sleep quality, and reduces cognitive performance the next day (Chang, Aeschbach, Duffy, and Czeisler, 2015).

Exposure to natural light from the sun during the daytime can help to counteract using a device with artificial light before bed (Rangtell, Ekstrand, Rapp, Lagermalm, Liethof, Bucaro, Lingfors, Broman, Schioth, and Benedict, 2016). Do me a favor, though. Invest in some blue light–blocking glasses and wear them for the last three hours before you go to bed.

Remember the herbal adaptogens I mentioned for help with hormone regulation? I swear by these at night and recommend taking them with magnesium glycinate. My favorite herbal adaptogen for sleep is the Ayurvedic herb Ashwagandha because it works so amazing for stress, brain health, and relaxation. If you react to nightshades, holy basil and rhodiola are great alternatives as well. Work with your practitioner to find the right blend of herbs for you.

Finally, it is important to sleep in total darkness. The tiniest bit of light alters our hormonal response to sleeping, and we sleep lighter and get less restorative sleep. I recommend using blackout curtains and wearing an eye mask to bed. Close your bedroom door, turn off your cell phone, and keep all lights out of the room. This ensures that our circadian rhythm can function properly.

Sleep cannot be underestimated, especially as we age. It becomes of utmost importance. It's time we start prioritizing sleep and see the amazing changes we experience in our health. Use these tried and true techniques; see if this makes a difference in your ability to fall asleep and stay asleep at night.

Chapter 10

ENSURING ADEQUATE SUN EXPOSURE

To trail our discussion on sleep, I wanted to touch upon the multiple benefits of sun exposure. Mainstream culture teaches us to fear the sun. We are warned over and over that the sun will give us cancer and age us. The mainstream medical community warns us to avoid the sun and cover up. Although extreme amounts of sun exposure may lead to certain types of skin cancer, research shows that the vitamin D we synthesize through sun exposure actually protects us from many forms of cancer.

Getting enough sun exposure each day is imperative to our health as we age. When we use high SPF sunscreens we not only block our photoreceptors (remember, they help to regulate our sleep cycle) but also inhibit the production of vitamin D. Many of the sunscreens out on the market contain neurotoxins and hormone disruptors that can contribute to hormone imbalance. Women who actively seek sunlight exposure regularly experience lower mortality than those who avoid the sun.

It's understandable to fear skin cancer, but we are not looking at the full picture here. Vitamin D plays many roles in our body and is essential for health. Evidence shows vitamin D from healthy sun exposure reduces the incidence of and increases the survival from many forms of cancer, including breast, colorectal, lung, ovarian, pancreatic, and prostate cancer. Vitamin D deficiency has been associated with a myriad of other health conditions including reproductive conditions, diabetes, multiple sclerosis, autoimmunity, and arthritis to name a few.

Every tissue in our body contains vitamin D receptors. The World Health Organization and the Surgeon General recommend avoiding the sun during peak times (10 a.m.–2 p.m.) and covering up any exposed areas with high SPF and protective clothing. However, this peak sun time is when vitamin D is most highly synthesized. Although neglecting the sun during this peak time may reduce the risk of certain skin melanomas, by completely avoiding any exposure during this time, we are blocking our ability to synthesize adequate vitamin D.

The sun is healing and relaxing for us! One of my favorite aspects of getting adequate sunlight is that the sun increases our feelings of well-being, boosts our immune system, and helps to relieve pain. UVB exposure actually helps to activate the hypothalamic pituitary axis, regulating homeostasis. This is that three-legged stool we discussed earlier that helps to keep our hormones in check.

Lack of sunlight contributes to cognitive impairments and depression. Melatonin and our feel good hormone, serotonin, are both regulated by the sun. Researchers found that cognitive functioning is also influenced by the sun, through the suprachiasmatic nuclei (SCN). We can literally alter our brain just by getting adequate sunlight.

How can we get adequate sunlight on our skin to support healthy hormones without getting burned?

- Go outside during peak sunlight hours (10 a.m.–2 p.m.) for about fifteen minutes (more or less, depending on the fairness of your skin). Gradually increase your sun exposure so you do not get a sunburn.
- Cover up with large hats and light-colored clothing rather than using potentially hormone-disruptive sunscreens.

- Eat healthy fats! This increases your intake of vitamins A, D, E, and K. I recommend lard, grass-fed butter, egg yolks, and liver. These nutrient-dense foods help to decrease inflammation associated with sunburns.
- Increase your intake of carotene- and lycopene-rich vegetables and fruits. These components help to protect the skin against damage from too much sun exposure.

Although getting burned by the sun can increase risk of melanoma, getting adequate sun exposure without burning decreases your risk of getting many different cancers. Don't avoid the sun; rather, focus on small amounts of sun exposure during peak times.

Afterword
IN CLOSING

As we age, we face many new challenges in our development. Our "second puberty" known as peri-menopause can feel like a turbulent time. My hope is that this book gives you some tools you can pull into your everyday life to help you grow physically, emotionally, and spiritually.

We never stop growing and changing. I like to think of each menstrual cycle as a mini birth and death. With each cycle we take a deeper and more meaningful look at our life and make changes where necessary. With every cycle we can begin anew. A new change, and a new chance. With turbulence comes deeper insights and new beginnings. We just have to accept all of it and accept all of ourselves as a whole being. We have to start facing our emotions, running toward them rather than away from them.

Let's take the time to honor our moods and stop

pushing them away. Let's nurture our body with sunlight, grounding, fresh air, and as much real food as possible. Let's move away from shallow, meaningless connections, and work to establish deeper intimacy with both ourselves and our partners. Let's prioritize our sleep, sexuality, and playfulness, and embrace all the good and bad this beautiful life continues to offer us as we enter a new phase in our lives.

THANK YOU!

Thank you so much for choosing to be on this journey with me. I am glad that you stopped by.

Please do not hesitate to connect with me if you have any questions come up about this book, or if you just want someone to chat with. I enjoy connecting with readers and would be happy to hear from you.

If you want more and would like to connect with me for future projects and happenings, just sign up on my blog to be notified of any pending book releases or updated content.

What are you waiting for?

Sign up now: http://primalmusings.com/timeforplay

Thanks again,
Kathryn Kos

A QUICK FAVOR PLEASE?

Before you go can I ask you for a quick favor?

Great, I knew I could count on you!

All I ask is that you please leave this book a review on Amazon. That's it! Easy, right?

Reviews are very important for authors like me, as they help us reach more people to sell more books, which, in turn enables me to write more books for you.

So please take a quick minute to go to Amazon and leave this book an honest review. I promise it doesn't take very long, and deeply impacts the work I can continue to do.

Thank you so much for reading, and for being part of the journey.

Until next time,
–Kathryn

REFERENCES

"About Binaural Beats: What Are Binaural Beats and How Do They Work?" Mindfit Hypnosis. April 24, 2018. https://www.mindfithypnosis.com/about-binaural-beats

Ballantyne, Sarah. *The Paleo Approach: Reverse Autoimmune Disease and Heal Your Body*. Las Vegas: Victory Belt Publishing, 2013.

Barth, Claudia, Arno Villringer, and Julia Sacher. "Sex Hormones Affect Neurotransmitters and Shape the Adult Female Brain during Hormonal Transition Periods." *Frontiers in Neuroscience* 9, no. 37 (2015). doi:10.3389/fnins.2015.00037.

Blessing, Esther M., Maria M. Steenkamp, Jorge Manzanares, and Charles R. Marmar. "Cannabidiol as a Potential Treatment for Anxiety Disorders." *Neurotherapeutics* 12, no. 4 (2015): 825-36. doi:10.1007/s13311-015-0387-1.

Brown, Dick, Ph.D., Gaetan Chevalier, Ph.D., and Michael Hill, B.S. "Pilot Study on the Effect of Grounding on Delayed-onset Muscle Soreness." *Journal of Alternative and Complementary*

Medicine 16, no. 3 (2010): 265-73. doi:10.1089/acm.2009.0399.

Brown, Stuart L., and Christopher C. Vaughan. *Play: How It Shapes the Brain, Opens the Imagination, and Invigorates the Soul.* New York: Avery, 2010.

Burstein, Sumner. "Cannabidiol (CBD) and Its Analogs: A Review of Their Effects on Inflammation." *Bioorganic & Medicinal Chemistry* 23, no. 7 (2015): 1377–385. doi:10.1016/j.bmc.2015.01.059.

Chandrasekhar, K., Jyoti Kapoor, and Sridhar Anishetty. "A Prospective, Randomized Double-blind, Placebo-controlled Study of Safety and Efficacy of a High-concentration Full-spectrum Extract of Ashwagandha Root in Reducing Stress and Anxiety in Adults." *Indian Journal of Psychological Medicine* 34, no. 3 (2012): 255-62. doi:10.4103/0253-7176.106022.

Chang, Anne-Marie, Daniel Aeschbach, Jeanne F. Duffy, and Charles A. Czeisler. "Evening Use of Light-emitting EReaders Negatively Affects Sleep, Circadian Timing, and Next-morning Alertness." *Proceedings of the National Academy of Sciences* 112, no. 4 (2014): 1232–237. doi:10.1073/pnas.1418490112.

Chevalier, Gaétan, Ph.D., and Stephen T. Sinatra, MD. "Emotional Stress, Heart Rate Variability, Grounding, and Improved Autonomic Tone: Clinical Applications." *Integrative Medicine* 10, no. 3 (2011): 16-21.

Chevalier, Gaétan, Stephen T. Sinatra, James L. Oschman, Karol Sokal, and Pawel Sokal. "Earthing: Health Implications of Reconnecting the Human Body to the Earth's Surface Electrons." *Journal of Environmental and Public Health* 2012 (2012): 1–8. doi:10.1155/2012/291541.

Dagher, Georges. "As Essential as Brushing Your Teeth: The Deep Squat." *Journal of Evolution and Health* 2, no. 1 (2017): 1–7. doi:10.15310/2334-3591.1052.

Dean, Carolyn. *The Magnesium Miracle*. New York: Ballantine Books, 2017.

Diederich, Kai, Anna Bastl, Heike Wersching, Anja Teuber, Jan-Kolja Strecker, Antje Schmidt, Jens Minnerup, and Wolf-Rüdiger Schäbitz. "Effects of Different Exercise Strategies and Intensities on Memory Performance and Neurogenesis." *Frontiers in Behavioral Neuroscience* 11 (2017). doi:10.3389/fnbeh.2017.00047.

"Dr. Jolene Brighten." Accessed August 20, 2018. https://drbrighten.com

Edwards, Darryl. *Animal Moves: How to Move Like an Animal to Get You Leaner, Fitter, Stronger, and Healthier for Life*. Explorer Publications, 2018.

Edwards, Darryl. "Play and the Feel Good Hormones." June 23, 2016. https://www.primalplay.com/blog/play-and-the-feel-good-hormones

Emmerich, Maria, and Craig Emmerich. *Keto: The Complete Guide to Success on the Ketogenic Diet, including Simplified Science and No-cook Meal Plans.* Las Vegas: Victory Belt Publishing, 2018.

Fear, Craig. *The 30 Day Heartburn Solution: A 3-step Nutrition Program to Stop Acid Reflux without Drugs.* Archangel Ink, 2015.

Ferretti, Gianluigi, Alessandra Felici, and Francesco Cognetti. "The Protective Side of Progesterone." *Breast Cancer Research* 9, no. 6 (2007). doi:10.1186/bcr1792.

"Find a Practitioner." https://www.ifm.org/find-a-practitioner

Fink, Julius, Naoki Kikuchi, and Koichi Nakazato. "Effects of Rest Intervals and Training Loads on Metabolic Stress and Muscle Hypertrophy." *Clinical Physiology and Functional Imaging* 38, no. 2 (2016): 261-68. doi:10.1111/cpf.12409.

Finn, Bridget, Ph.D. Telephone interview by author.

Gaudreau, Stephanie. Telephone interview by author.

Ghaly, Maurice, and Dale Teplitz. "The Biologic Effects of Grounding the Human Body during Sleep as Measured by Cortisol Levels and Subjective Reporting of Sleep, Pain, and Stress." *The Journal of Alternative and Complementary Medicine* 10, no. 5 (2004): 767–76. doi:10.1089/1075553042476696.

Gilbert, Elizabeth. *Eat, Pray, Love: One Woman's Search for Everything across Italy, India, and Indonesia.* New York: Penguin, 2007.

Holland, Julie. *Moody Bitches: The Truth about the Drugs You're Not Taking, the Sleep You're Missing, the Sex You're Not Having, and What's Really Making You Crazy*. Penguin, 2015.

Ignacio, Daniele Leão, Diego H. Da S. Silvestre, João Paulo Albuquerque Cavalcanti-De-Albuquerque, Ruy Andrade Louzada, Denise P. Carvalho, and João Pedro Werneck-De-Castro. "Thyroid Hormone and Estrogen Regulate Exercise-induced Growth Hormone Release." *Plos One* 10, no. 4 (2015). doi:10.1371/journal.pone.0122556.

Kahn, Suliman, Pengfei Duan, Lunguang Yao, and Hongwei Hou, "Shiftwork-Mediated Disruptions of Circadian Rhythms and Sleep Homeostasis Cause Serious Health Problems." *International Journal of Genomics.* Volume 2018. https://doi.org/10.1155/2018/8576890

Kashani, L., M.D., R. Hajighaee, Ph.D., and S. Akhondzadeh, Ph.D. "Herbal Medicine in the Treatment of Premenstrual Syndromes." *Journal of Medicinal Plants* 10, no. 37 (2011): 1–5. http://jmp.ir/article-1-227-en.pdf

Katz, Sandor E. *Wild Fermentation: The Flavor, Nutrition, and Craft of Live-culture Foods.* White River Junction, VT: Chelsea Green Publishing, 2008.

Kozaki, Tomoaki, Naohiro Toda, Hiroki Noguchi, and Akira Yasukouchi. "Effects of Different Light Intensities in the Morning on Dim Light Melatonin Onset." *Journal of PHYSIOLOGICAL*

ANTHROPOLOGY 30, no. 3 (2011): 97-102. doi:10.2114/jpa2.30.97.

Maté, Gabor. *When the Body Says No: Understanding the Stress-disease Connection*. John Wiley & Sons, 2011.

McLachlan, J. A. "Environmental Signaling: From Environmental Estrogens to Endocrine-disrupting Chemicals and beyond." *Andrology* 4, no. 4 (2016): 684–94. doi:10.1111/andr.12206.

Muhammad, Aslam, and Nasir Ali. "Antidepressant-like Activity of Ethanol Extract of Ganoderma Lucidum (reishi) in Mice." *International Journal of Medical Research & Health Sciences* 6, no. 5 (2017): 55–58. https://www.ijmrhs.com/medical-research/antidepressantlike-activity-of-ethanol-extract-of-ganoderma-lucidum-reishi-in-mice.pdf

Ober, Clinton, Stephen T. Sinatra, and Martin Zucker. *Earthing: The Most Important Health Discovery Ever?* Sydney: Basic Health Publications, 2010.

Oschman, James L. "Can Electrons Act as Antioxidants? A Review and Commentary." *The Journal of Alternative and Complementary Medicine* 13, no. 9 (2007): 955–67. doi:10.1089/acm.2007.7048.

Oschman, James L. "Perspective: Assume a Spherical Cow: The Role of Free or Mobile Electrons in Bodywork, Energetic and Movement Therapies." *Journal of Bodywork and Movement Therapies* 12, no. 1 (2008): 40-57. doi:10.1016/j.jbmt.2007.08.002.

Oschman, James, Gaetan Chevalier, and Richard Brown. "The Effects of Grounding (earthing) on Inflammation, the Immune Response, Wound Healing, and Prevention and Treatment of Chronic Inflammatory and Autoimmune Diseases." *Journal of Inflammation Research*, 2015, 83. doi:10.2147/jir.s69656.

Panos Egglezos. March 11, 2012. Accessed August 20, 2018. https://www.youtube.com/watch?v=Cfk2IX1ZdbI

"Perimenopause." June 2, 2018. Accessed August 20, 2018. https://www.webmd.com/menopause/guide/guide-perimenopause

Permutter, David. *Grain Brain: The Surprising Truth about Wheat, Carbs, and Sugar—Your Brain's Silent Killers.* S.l.: Little, Brown, 2013.

Posaci, Cemal, Oktay Erten, Ali Üren, and Berrin Acar. "Plasma Copper, Zinc and Magnesium Levels in Patients with Premenstrual Tension Syndrome." *Acta Obstetricia Et Gynecologica Scandinavica* 73, no. 6 (1994): 452-55. doi:10.3109/00016349409013429.

Prior, Jerilynn C. "Ovarian Aging and the Perimenopausal Transition: The Paradox of Endogenous Ovarian Hyperstimulation." *Endocrine* 26, no. 3 (2005): 297–300. doi:10.1385/endo:26:3:297.

Rångtell, Frida H., Emelie Ekstrand, Linnea Rapp, Anna Lagermalm, Lisanne Liethof, Marcela O. Búcaro, David Lingfors, Jan-Erik Broman, Helgi B. Schiöth, and Christian Benedict. "Two Hours of Evening Reading on a Self-luminous Tablet vs. Reading a Physical Book Does Not Alter Sleep after Daytime Bright Light Exposure." *Sleep Medicine* 23 (2016): 111-18. doi:10.1016/j.sleep.2016.06.016.

Ruiz, Don Miguel. *The Mastery of Love: A Practical Guide to the Art of Relationship*. Amber-Allen Publishing, 2011.

Sanfilippo, Diane, Bill Staley, and Robb Wolf. *Practical Paleo: A Customized Approach to Health and a Whole-foods Lifestyle*. Las Vegas: Victory Belt Publishing, 2012.

Seifert-Klauss, Vanadin, and Jerilynn C. Prior. "Progesterone and Bone: Actions Promoting Bone Health in Women." *Journal of Osteoporosis* 2010 (2010): 1–18. doi:10.4061/2010/845180.

"Shine the Light on Blue Light." http://www.bluelightexposed.com/#where-is-the-increased-exposure-to-blue-light-coming-from

Si, Daowen, Juan Li, Jiang Liu, Xiaoyin Wang, Zifeng Wei, Qingyou Tian, Haitao Wang, and Gang Liu. "Progesterone Protects Blood-brain Barrier Function and Improves Neurological Outcome following Traumatic Brain Injury in Rats." *Experimental and Therapeutic Medicine* 8, no. 3 (2014): 1010-014. doi:10.3892/etm.2014.1840.

Sisson, Mark. *The New Primal Blueprint: Reprogram Your Genes for Effortless Weight Loss, Vibrant Health, and*

Boundless Energy. Oxnard, CA: Primal Nutrition, Incorporated, 2016.

Sokal, Karol, and Pawel Sokal. "Earthing the Human Body Influences Physiologic Processes." *The Journal of Alternative and Complementary Medicine* 17, no. 4 (2011): 301–08. doi:10.1089/acm.2010.0687.

Thomas, Peter, and Yefei Pang. "Protective Actions of Progesterone in the Cardiovascular System: Potential Role of Membrane Progesterone Receptors (mPRs) in Mediating Rapid Effects." *Steroids* 78, no. 6 (2013): 583–88. doi:10.1016/j.steroids.2013.01.003.

Vahratian, Anjel. "Sleep Duration and Quality Among Women Aged 40–59, by Menopausal Status." *NCHS Data Brief*, no. 286 (2017).

Watson, Cheryl S., Guangzhen Hu, and Adriana A. Paulucci-Holthauzen. "Rapid Actions of Xenoestrogens Disrupt Normal Estrogenic Signaling." *Steroids* 81 (2014): 36–42. doi:10.1016/j.steroids.2013.11.006.

"Ways Sitting Is Shortening Your Life." July 31, 2015. https://www.theactivetimes.com/ways-sitting-shortening-your-life

Whitfield, Charles L., and Cardwell C. Nuckols. *Healing the Child Within: Discovery and Recovery for Adult Children of Dysfunctional Families*. Deerfield Beach, FL: Health Communications, 2015.

ABOUT THE AUTHOR

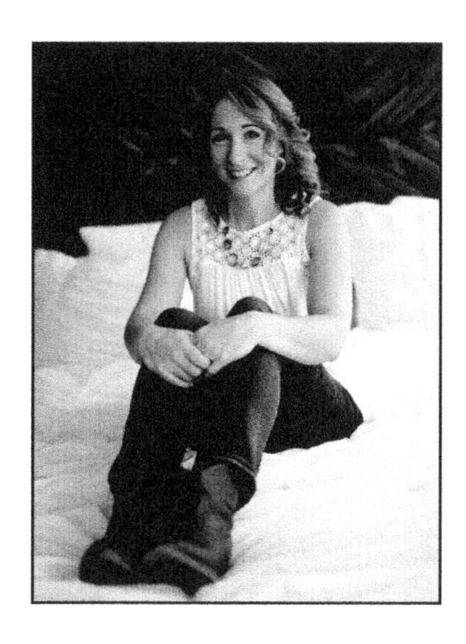

Kathryn Kos is an experienced Nutritional Therapy Practitioner with an M.Ed. in Rehabilitation Counseling. Her focus is on helping women overcome emotional and hormonal imbalance, creating diet and fitness plans that lead to total wellness while fostering healthy sleep and sexuality. After years of working with clients, Kathryn saw a need for more widespread information about the effects of perimenopause and consequently wrote her first book, *Forties on Fire: Rediscover Your Sexuality, Learn to Honor Your Moods, and Thrive Throughout Your 40s and Beyond.*

Kathryn is an HSP (highly sensitive person) and among the 1% as an INFJ on Meyers Briggs (MBTI). She is mom to two boys and longs to inspire people to break free from their thought patterns and continuously learn and grown as humans, while striving for more deep, meaningful, and healing connections with each other. She encourages women to value their strength, true inner beauty, and vitality in their 40's and beyond. She lives in Upstate NY, where she enjoys hiking the high peaks with her dog Sunflower.

Made in the USA
Middletown, DE
09 March 2019